Blood Pressure Solution

The Ultimate Beginner's Guide

30 Proven Natural Super Foods to Control & Lower Your High Blood Pressure

By *Ethan Daniel*

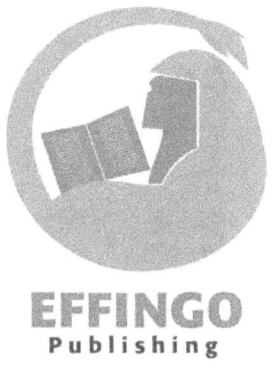

For more great books, visit:

EffingoPublishing.com

Download another book for Free

We want to thank you for purchasing this book and offer you another book (just as long and valuable as this book), "Health & Fitness Mistakes You Don't Know You're Making," completely free.

Visit the link below to sign up and receive it:

www.effingopublishing.com/gift

In this book, we will break down the most common health & fitness mistakes, you are probably committing right now, and will reveal how you can quickly get in the best shape of your life!

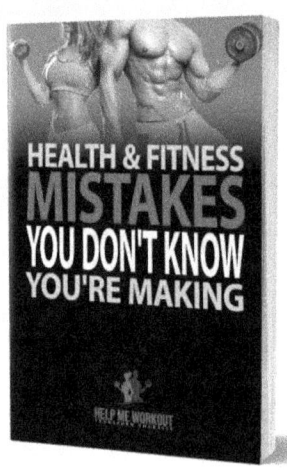

In addition to this valuable gift, you will also have an opportunity to get our new books for free, enter giveaways, and receive other useful emails from us. Again, visit the link to sign up:

www.effingopublishing.com/gi

TABLE OF CONTENTS

Introduction 7

Chapter 1: What is high blood pressure, causes, and diseases associated with it? 9

Signs and Symptoms 9

Risk Factors of High Blood Pressure 11

chapter 2: Benefits of Reducing and controlling blood pressure...22

Improve your heart health 22

Chapter 3: Natural superfoods to eat when you have high blood pressure 27

Chapter 4: What not to eat when you have high blood pressure...38

Chapter 5: High blood pressure solution vs. Weight loss – What's the Difference?........................45

Maximize Protein 46

Chapter 6: Effective meal plan to help you reduce and control high blood pressure 50

Day 1 50

Day 2: 53

Day 3 57

Day 4 59

Day 5 63

Day 6 67

Day 7 70

Day 8 73

Day 9 78

Day 10 80

Day 11 82

Day 12 84

Day 13 89

Day 14 93

Day 15 97

Day 16 101

Day 17 104

Day 18 107

Day 19 109

Day 20 111

Day 21 113

Day 22 115

Day 23 117

Day 24 121

Day 25 125

Day 26 128

Day 27 131

Day 28 135

Day 29 137

Day 30 140

Chapter 7: Strategies to get started on lower blood pressure meal diet 142

Chapter 8: Other lifestyle changes to help you reduce blood pressure without medication 144

Conclusion 146

Final Words 147

About the Co-Author 148

INTRODUCTION

High blood pressure is a significant public health challenge these days due to its high prevalence, and the concomitant increase in the risk of other high blood pressure-related complications. Since there are few signs, this potential fatal health issue often goes unnoticed.

While high blood pressure usually doesn't show symptoms for the first 10-20 years, it slowly but surely damages the arteries and strains the heart. This is why this condition is called the "silent killer." Prolonged high blood pressure accelerates arteriosclerosis, which is the leading cause of vascular disease, stroke, heart failure, and renal failure.

Advanced warning signs include rapid pulse, dizziness, vision disturbances, sweating, headache, and shortness of breath. It can be because of age, diet, obesity, stress, smoking, race, or heredity. The good thing is there are natural solutions without medication that you can maximize. Learn more about the causes and diseases associated with it, natural foods to help control high blood pressure, and effective meal plan for you.

Also, before you get started, I recommend you **joining our email newsletter** to receive updates on any upcoming new book releases or promotions. You can sign-up for free, and as a bonus, you will receive a gift. Our "*Health & Fitness Mistakes You Don't Know You're Making*" book! This book has been written to demystify, expose the top do's and don'ts and to finally equip you with the information you need to get in the best shape of your life. Due to the overwhelming amount of misinformation and lies told by magazines and self-proclaimed "gurus, " it's becoming harder and harder to get reliable information to get in shape. As opposed to having to go through dozens of biased, unreliable, and untrustworthy sources to get your health & fitness information. Everything you need to help you has been broken down in this book for you to easily follow and to immediately get results to achieve your desired fitness goals in the shortest amount of time.

Once again, to join our free email newsletter and to receive a free copy of this valuable book, please visit the link and signup now: **www.effingopublishing.com/gift.**

CHAPTER 1: WHAT IS HIGH BLOOD PRESSURE, CAUSES, AND DISEASES ASSOCIATED WITH IT?

High blood pressure is a condition that happens when your blood pressure increase to unhealthy levels. Blood pressure is measured with the blood passing through your blood vessels, and the resistance the blood meets while the heart is pumping. Having narrow arteries increase this resistance, and thus, a higher blood pressure. Through time, higher blood pressure can cause other health issues.

You can have high blood pressure for years without having any symptoms. Even if it is asymptomatic, the damage to your heart and blood vessels continues and can be detected. Over the years, it generally develops and affects nearly everyone eventually. The good thing is it can be identified quickly, and once you know you have high blood pressure, you can work on controlling it.

Signs and Symptoms

High blood pressure doesn't cause any symptoms, which is why it is called "the silent killer." People typically don't know that they suffer from it until they measure their blood pressure. At times, people with elevated blood pressure may develop other diseases and complications because the organs are stressed when exposed to high pressures. Here are the signs and symptoms that you have high blood pressure:

- **Brain symptoms for high blood pressure**
    1. Blurred vision

2. Dizziness

3. Nausea and vomiting

4. Headache

- **Heart symptoms for high blood pressure**

    1. Weakness

    2. Chest pain

    3. Nausea and vomiting

    4. Shortness of breath

- **Chronic high blood pressure symptoms**
    1. Kidney failure
    2. Heart failure
    3. Aneurysms (outpouchings of the aorta)
    4. Transient ischemic attack or mini-stroke
    5. Peripheral arterial disease (pain on the leg when walking)
    6. Heart attack
    7. Eye damage with progressive vision loss

It is vital to realize that high blood pressure can be asymptomatic and thus, unrecognized for years. However, it causes progressive damage to your heart, blood vessels and other organs.

Risk Factors of High Blood Pressure

There are variables and factors, which can put you at risk for developing high blood pressure. However, understanding these risk factors can be helpful and can increase awareness and prevention.

- **Hereditary and physical risk factors for high blood pressure**
    1. **Age:** The risk of high blood pressure increases as we age. As we age, our blood vessels gradually lose some elastic quality, and this is a massive contributor to elevated blood pressure.

2. **Gender:** While age is one of the primary risk factors for high blood pressure, men are more likely to get this condition at the age of 64. On the other hand, women are more likely to develop high blood pressure after 65 years old.

3. **Family history:** If your parents and other direct family members (and close blood relatives) have high blood pressure, you are more likely to get the condition as well.

4. **Race:** African-Americans are more likely to develop high blood pressure as compared to other racial backgrounds in the United States. It is particularly common among African heritage and often develops at an earlier age.

5. **Chronic kidney disease:** High blood pressure may also occur as a result of kidney disease and may cause even more kidney damage.

- **Changeable risk factors for high blood pressure**

    1. **Obesity or overweight:** Carrying too much weight can put an additional strain on your heart and the circulatory system, which causes serious health problems. This is because the more weight you have, the more you need to supply oxygen and nutrients to your tissues. If the blood volume that is circulating through your blood vessels increases, the pressure on your artery walls does the same. It may also increase your risk of diabetes and cardiovascular disease.

    2. **Sleep apnea:** Obstructive sleep apnea can increase the chance of developing high blood pressure. It is common in people who have resistant hypertension.

    3. **High cholesterol:** More than half of people with high blood pressure also have high cholesterol.

    4. **Physical inactivity:** Not getting enough physical activity as part of your lifestyle is also a contributor to increased blood pressure. People who are not active physically tend to have higher heart rates, and the higher your heart rate, the harder your heart needs to work with every contraction; thereby, the stronger the force on your arteries. It is also a risk factor in getting overweight. Doing some physical activity is excellent for your heart and circulatory system, and prevents or controls high blood pressure.

5. **Smoking and using tobacco:** Smoking can cause temporary high blood pressure and can cause damage to arteries. This can cause your arteries to narrow and increases the risk of heart disease. Aside from that, secondhand smoking or exposure to other people's smoke can also increase the risk of heart disease for non-smokers.

6. **Drinking too much alcohol:** Heavy use or regular alcohol intake may cause many health problems, including stroke, heart failure, and arrhythmia (irregular heartbeat). It can cause a dramatic increase in blood pressure and can increase the risk of obesity, cancer, and alcoholism.

7. **Stress:** Stress is not necessarily a bad thing, but too much stress may be another contributor to elevated blood pressure. Furthermore, too much stress may encourage behaviors that increase blood pressure, such as drinking alcohol or using tobacco more than usual, poor diet, and physical inactivity.

8. **Diabetes:** Most people who have diabetes also develop high blood pressure.

9. **Unhealthy food:** It is crucial to have proper nutrition from different sources. A diet with high salt consumptions and high calories, along with sugar, trans, and saturated fat, carries more risks of high blood pressure. Alternatively, having a healthy diet and food options can help in controlling your blood pressure.

Pregnancy can also be a contributor to high blood pressure. And even though this condition is most common in adults, children may also be at risk. For some children, increased blood pressure is caused by heart or kidney problems. For a growing number of children, poor lifestyle habits like obesity, unhealthy diet, and lack of exercise can increase the risk of high blood pressure.

Complications

The excessive pressure on your artery walls caused by high blood pressure can cause damage to your blood vessels and body organs. The higher your blood pressure, and longer it goes uncontrolled, the greater the complications.

- **Damage to your heart**

    High blood pressure causes many heart problems, and having awareness will help control causes.

    1. **Heart failure:** Through time, the strain on your heart because of high blood pressure can cause weakened and inefficient heart muscle. Your overwhelmed heart eventually starts failing. Damage from heart attacks is another contributor to this problem.

    2. **Coronary artery disease:** Damaged and narrowed arteries caused by high blood pressure have difficulty supplying blood to your heart. If the blood cannot flow to your heart freely, it may cause you irregular heart rhythms, chest pain, and heart attack.

    3. **Enlarged left heart:** When you have high blood pressure, your heart is forced to work harder to pump blood to the rest of your body. This causes thickened left ventricle, thus, result in an increased risk of heart failure, heart attack, and even sudden cardiac death.

- **Damage to your arteries**

    Healthy arteries are elastic, reliable, and flexible, with inner lining being smooth, allowing blood to flow freely. Thus, it supplies oxygen and nutrients to vital organs. However, high blood pressure increases the pressure of blood flowing through your arteries gradually and causes damage to your arteries.

1. **Aneurysm:** Through time, the consistent pressure of blood moving through a damaged or weakened artery may cause a wall section to enlarge and form a bulge or aneurysm. This can result in rupture and life-threatening internal bleeding. This artery condition may develop in any artery but most common in the largest artery.

2. **Narrowed and damaged arteries:** High blood pressure can damage the inner lining cells of your arteries. When fats from your diet enter your bloodstream, they can be accumulated in the damaged arteries. Your artery walls then become less elastic, which limits blood from flowing throughout your body.

- **Damage to your kidney**

    Kidneys are filtering the excess waste and fluid from your blood, which requires healthy blood vessels to function. High blood pressure can damage the blood vessels leading to your kidneys and even inside your kidneys. It can also worsen the damage if you have diabetes.

    1. **Kidney failure:** High blood pressure is one of the most common causes of kidney failure. Blood vessels being damaged prevent kidneys from filtering the blood waster effectively, which allows dangerous fluid and waste levels to accumulate. You might be required to undergo kidney transplantation and dialysis because of it.

    2. **Glomerulosclerosis (kidney scarring):** This kidney damage happens when the little blood vessels within the kidney become scarred and cannot filter waste and fluid from your blood effectively and may lead to kidney failure.

- **Damage to your brain**

    Your brain requires a nourishing blood supply to work correctly, but high blood pressure can cause many problems to the brain.

    1. **Transient ischemic attack:** It is like a mini-stroke, which temporarily disrupts the blood supply to your brain. Hardened blood clots or arteries caused by increased blood pressure can cause a transient ischemic attack

and is usually a warning that you are at risk of a full-blown stroke.

2. **Stroke:** Stroke can happen when part of your brain is deprived of nutrients and oxygen, which causes the brain cell to die. Damaged blood vessels caused by high blood pressure can rupture, leak, or narrow. Also, an increase in blood pressure may cause blood clots to form in the arteries and to your brain, which blocks the flow of blood. This results in a stroke.

3. **Dementia:** Blocked or narrowed arteries may provide limited blood flow to your brain, which leads to a particular type of dementia called vascular dementia. You can also get vascular dementia with a stroke interrupting the blood flow to the brain.

4. **Mild cognitive impairment:** It is generally caused by changes in memory and understanding due to dementia.

- **Damage to your eyes**

    High blood pressure can damage even the delicate tiny blood vessels that supply blood to your eyes.

    1. **Retinopathy:** Retinopathy is damage to your retina, which can lead to eye bleeding, blurred, or even complete vision loss. You are at even greater risk if you also have diabetes aside from high blood pressure.

    2. **Optic neuropathy:** If the flow of blood is blocked, it can also damage the optic nerve, which results in eye-bleeding and even loss of vision.

    3. **Choroidopathy:** Fluid buildup under the retina may result in distorted vision.

- **Sexual dysfunction**

    It has been prevalent in men with ages 50 and up to be unable to maintain or have an erection. However, men with high blood pressure are even more likely to experience dysfunction. This is because of the limited blood flowing to the penis.

    Moreover, women may also experience sexual dysfunction due to high blood pressure. Limited blood flow to the vagina may lead to decrease arousal or sexual desire, difficulty attaining orgasm, or vaginal dryness.

- **High blood pressure emergencies**

    Increased blood pressure is generally a chronic condition that causes damage throughout the years.

However, blood pressure sometimes increases so quickly and even severely that it becomes a medical emergency. It could require immediate treatment or hospitalization.

1. Stroke
2. Heart attack
3. Personality changes, irritability, trouble concentrating, memory loss, and/or progressive loss of consciousness
4. Blindness
5. Sudden loss of kidney function
6. Chest pain
7. Severe damage to the main artery
8. Complications in pregnancy (eclampsia or pre-eclampsia)

CHAPTER 2: BENEFITS OF REDUCING AND CONTROLLING BLOOD PRESSURE

Blood pressure is required to be high enough to give the organs the blood and nutrients that they need without being too high to the point of damaging blood vessels. As such, our bodies need to maintain and control blood pressure, keeping it at an average level.

High blood pressure is a dangerous condition that needs to be treated appropriately. As time passes by, once damage already occurred to the heart and other organs, it usually cannot be reversed anymore. Uncontrolled high blood pressure damages, mainly the heart and other organs. It accelerates the hardening of arteries and the build-up of cholesterol-laden plaques on arterial walls.

Improve your heart health

High blood pressure puts a strain in the heart, which results in an increased risk of peripheral artery disease, angina, heart failure, heart attack, and coronary artery disease. Through time, the heart becomes damaged and result in an enlarged heart. When it is damaged, the body cannot undo it anymore. With high blood pressure, you are 3x more likely to get cardiovascular heart complications.

A healthful eating plan will help in improving your heart health. Include vegetables, whole grains, limited lean meat, seafood, non-fat dairy products, beans, and fruits in your diet plan. Additionally, it is essential to control your weight and reduce stress. Some helpful tips include improving your sleep, body composition, and your ability to perform daily activities. Make sure to lower your blood sugar and lower your risk of type II diabetes.

Reduce the risk of stroke

Potential damage to blood vessels caused by higher blood pressure contributes to ischemic stroke. This is another reason why lowering your blood pressure helps in reducing the risk of stroke, along with other complications associated with stroke.

Reduce your salt intake to no more than 1500mg per day, which is equivalent to a half teaspoon. Another helpful food tip is to avoid food that has high cholesterol, such as ice cream, burgers, and cheese. It is also advisable to eat 4-5 cups of vegetables and fruits daily, with added fish 2-3x per week and a serving of low-fat dairy and whole grains several days a week. Go for a lose-weight diet plan, too.

Improve your vision

It is essential to lower down your blood pressure because uncontrolled blood pressure may also result in hypertensive retinopathy – a condition affecting the retina of the eye. The only treatment for this disease is to lower and maintain your blood pressure levels. This means that if you have a hypertensive stroke, your vision will also be at risk. Strokes have an effect on the optic nerve and the parts of the brain that is mainly responsible for processing the things you see.

Eating carrots is good for your eyes, as it is rich in vitamin A, which is a vital nutrient for your vision. But vitamin A is not the only nutrient needed to improve your vision; it is also advisable to include foods that are high in vitamin E, vitamin C, zinc, and copper to your diet plan.

Your biggest challenge is macular degeneration, so it is also helpful to take anti-oxidants like carrots, sweet potatoes, pumpkins, eggs, and dark green vegetables. Fish is also good for the eyes, so eat food with fatty acid. Cold fish like wild salmon, cod, and mackerel help in strengthening cell membranes, and these also contain DHA.

Protect your kidney

Lowering and/or maintaining a healthy blood pressure level can help prevent this vicious cycle and lessen the chance of complete kidney failure. Eat healthily and keep your weight in check, as it is a great help in preventing heart disease, diabetes, and other conditions linked to chronic kidney disease. Helpful tips start with reducing your salt intake. Follow the recommended sodium intake of about 5-6g daily. To be able to decrease your intake of salt, try to limit the amount of restaurant food and processed food, and add some alternative spices instead when you are cooking dishes. Prepare the food yourself with fresh ingredients.

Furthermore, drinking lots of fluid helps your kidney in clearing urea, sodium, and even the other toxins in your body. This results in a radically reduced risk of chronic kidney complications. Excessive fluid can also be harmful, so make sure to take the right level of fluid intake daily, depending on several factors like your exercise, other health condition, gender, climate, breastfeeding, and/or pregnancy.

Improve your quality of life and increase the life span

There are about 1000 people who were dying from high blood pressure just in the entirety of the United States every year. 50% died from heart disease, heart failure, and 40% from diabetes. High blood pressure is also a leading risk for fetal and maternal death in pregnancy, renal failure, and dementia. By lowering your blood pressure to an average level, you are 25% less likely to be at risk of death due to complications of this condition, mainly from cardiovascular disease.

Lower pocket expenses

When you reduce and maintain healthy blood pressure, you also save money. This is because having high blood pressure condition costs nearly 50 billion dollars per year. You are not only saving money but also time you could spend in the hospital. You will be able to avoid maintenance medicine, dialysis, treatments, and schedules. It gives you more chance to focus on using that money for better use and other investments.

Investments in prevention are cost-saving

Lowering and maintaining healthy blood pressure is cost-saving by improving diet and physical activity. It also allows you to make healthy choices.

There are only about 52% of people, primarily adults, who have their blood pressure level under control. You may start managing your blood pressure today by making small changes in your daily life, including the way you eat.

CHAPTER 3: NATURAL SUPERFOODS TO EAT WHEN YOU HAVE HIGH BLOOD PRESSURE

Changes in diet can significantly lower blood pressure levels. There are effective foods that can reduce blood pressure, both instantly and in the long term. Dietary change results in a reduction of a few points in just two weeks. Through time, the top number of your blood pressure level could be lowered down by 8-14 points, resulting in a significant difference in your health risks.

1. **Banana:** Banana contains lots of potassium, a mineral that plays a vital role in maintaining blood pressure level. Potassium lowers the effects of sodium, resulting in tension alleviation in the walls of blood vessels. Eating foods that are rich in potassium is better than taking supplements. Put a sliced banana in your oatmeal or cereal for a potassium-rich addition. You may also choose one to go along with a boiled egg for a quick breakfast or snack.

2. **Oatmeal:** Oatmeal fits the bill for a low-sodium, low-fat, and high-fiber way of reducing your blood pressure level. Eating oatmeal for breakfast is an excellent way to fuel up your day. On the other hand, overnight oats are also a great breakfast option. Soak ½ cup of rolled oats and ½ cup of nut milk in a jar. You can eat them in the morning and add some cinnamon, berries, and granola to taste. Moreover, the fiber can help you maintain healthy body weight

and prevent obesity, which is a risk factor for high blood pressure.

3. **Flaxseed:** You may also stir some flax into your favorite morning oatmeal or smoothie. Flaxseed is an excellent source of fiber and omega-3 fatty acids, which mainly lower inflammation throughout the body. It helps improve the health of your heart and circulatory system. Omega-3 has a significant effect on lower diastolic and systolic blood pressure.

4. **Berries:** Strawberries and blueberries contain antioxidant compounds called anthocyanins – a type of flavonoid. Consuming these compounds have a significant impact on the prevention of high blood pressure. On the other hand, aside from flavonoids, berries are also high in fiber and loaded with resveratrol, which is also useful for blood pressure reduction. The good thing is that it is easy to add to your diet. You can put them on your granola or cereal in the morning, or you may keep frozen berries on hand for a healthy dessert.

5. **Onion:** It may not be suitable for your breath, but it cannot be beaten when it comes to lowering blood pressure. This is because onion is a great source of quercetin, and it has been found effective in the reduction of blood pressure in obese and overweight. You may try making your onion less pungent by sauteing them in olive oil for a sweeter flavor and omega-3 fatty acid.

6. **Olive oil:** Olive oil is an example of healthy fat, which contains polyphenols. It helps lower blood pressure levels because it is an inflammation-fighting compound. It helps specifically elderly patients who have systolic blood pressure. Also, it can meet your 2-3 everyday servings of fat as part of the high-blood-pressure diet. It is also a great alternative to butter, canola oil, or commercial salad dressing.

7. **Dark chocolate:** Eating dark chocolate helps in lowering your risk of cardiovascular disease. It contains more than 60% cocoa solids and has less sugar as compared to regular chocolate. It is rich in antioxidants called flavanols, which is a compound that helps blood vessels to be more elastic. It will result in an improved flow of blood to the heart and brain, making blood platelets less sticky. It also reduces the risk of heart disease. You may eat it with fruits like raspberries, strawberries, or blueberries as a healthy dessert, or add it to your yogurt. Stick to one ounce of dark chocolate per day and make sure it has 60-70% cocoa.

8. **Pomegranates:** This fruit may be small, but it has a lot of serious nutritional compounds. The juice from the seed is polyphenol-rich, which is an antioxidant with many benefits alone. It helps in the prevention of cancer. Pomegranate juice has a significant effect on reduced systolic and diastolic blood pressure through time, even when consumed in small amounts. The juice can be tasty with a healthy breakfast. Make sure to check the sugar content in store-bought juices, as the added sugars may negate the health benefits. Or you may enjoy it whole.

9. **Pistachios:** Pistachio is a healthy nut that helps decrease high blood pressure. Including this nut in a

moderate-fat diet can lower down blood pressure during times of stress. It helps the brain to stay sharp. This is because a compound in the nuts lowers down the blood vessel's tightness. You can incorporate pistachio in your diet by adding them to pesto sauces, crusts, and salads, or you can eat them plain as a snack.

10. **Watermelon:** It is a good source of lycopene and vitamin C, which contributes significantly to lowering blood pressure levels. Also, it contains an amino acid called citrulline, which helps in controlling and maintaining blood pressure. Citrulline helps the body to produce nitric oxide – a gas that relaxes blood vessels and encourages arteries flexibility, especially in the ankles and arms. These effects help in the blood flow. And has a high impact on overweight people both to manage blood pressure and stress. To improve watermelon intake, add it to smoothies and salads, or enjoy within a chilled watermelon soup, or plain after lunch/snack.

11. **Kale:** It contains beta-carotene, quercetin, and vitamin C, which has been effective in reducing blood pressure naturally. It also contains magnesium and potassium, which are vital minerals to control blood pressure. A potassium-rich diet helps the body to become more efficient at flushing out excess sodium (that can increase the blood pressure). On the other hand, magnesium helps in promoting a healthy flow of blood. To consume a daily dose of this green vegetable, you may stir it into stews and curries, or bake a batch of kale chips.

12. **Skim milk:** A glass of milk provides an excellent service of both vitamin D and calcium, which are nutrients essential for lowering blood pressure by as much as 3-10%. Those percentages may not sound impressive, but they could be translated into a 15% reduction in the risk of a heart attack. Higher dietary intake of calcium helps lower diastolic and systolic blood pressure. Try incorporating almond slivers, fruits, and granola into your yogurt for additional heart-healthy benefits.

13. **Apple:** An apple a day indeed keeps the doctor away, specifically for those who have high blood pressure. Aside from the 4.5 grams of blood pressure-lowering fiber, apple also has quercetin that is a helpful antihypertensive remedy. It is an excellent alternative for kiwi.

14. **Kiwi:** It is another fruit with a positive effect on lowering blood pressure levels. Eating three kiwis a day over eight weeks has a positive result in lower blood pressure. Another blood pressure-lowering content of kiwi is vitamin C. You can add this fruit to your lunch or smoothies.

15. **Garlic:** Garlic is a natural antifungal and antibiotic food and has a primary active ingredient called allicin, which has other health benefits. Garlic improves nitric oxide production, relaxing the smooth muscles, and dilating the blood vessels. These changes are helpful in decreased blood pressure levels. It can reduce both diastolic and systolic blood pressure in hypertensive people. Additionally, garlic enhances the flavor of many savory meals, including omelets, stir-fries, and soups.

So it is not hard to add to your diet. You may use garlic instead of salt to promote heart health benefits further.

16. **Salmon (and other fish with omega-3 fatty acid**: While fatty foods may seem like they do not have a place in high blood pressure-lowering meal plan, salmon specifically is one major exception to that rule. This is because salmon is filled with heart-healthy omega-3 fatty acids – helpful in reducing inflammation, thus, lowering the risk of heart disease. This results in getting the blood pressure into a healthy level. Supplementing your body with omega-3 reduces blood pressure also on older patients and patients with hypertension. The good thing is that it is easy to cook. Place a salmon fillet in parchment paper and season with lemon, herbs, and olive oil. Bake the fish in a preheated oven at 450 degrees F for 12 to 15 minutes.

17. **Apricots**: Lower your risk of chronic disease and control blood pressure level by making apricots a staple in your diet. Apricot is loaded with carotene, which is one of the critical nutrients needed in healthier blood pressure. It also provides fiber that also has a significant effect on reducing blood pressure. You may toss some on your favorite salad, or you may eat dried apricots for a snack. It can even be added to your smoothie.

18. **Egg**: While egg has had a bad reputation in the past due to its cholesterol content, but the protein it contains helps improve both the cholesterol and blood pressure level while keeping you satisfied. A diet high in protein doesn't only help reduce blood pressure naturally but also promotes weight loss. Just make sure not to add some wrong condiments to

your egg-based breakfast to prevent destruction on the health benefits. The high salt content in hot sauce and sugar in ketchup may lower the effects of egg in reducing blood pressure levels.

19. **Spinach**: Making spinach a part of your blood pressure-lowering routine is an excellent choice as it contains magnesium and potassium to control blood pressure to a reasonable level. It also has beta-carotene, vitamin C, and fiber, which then again helpful for lowering blood pressure. It is an alternative for your other veggie options like kale. You can blend this vegetable with nut milk and banana for a healthy, sweet green juice.

20. **Tomato**: A little tomato on your blood-pressure-lowering diet is helpful. Aside from the high content of quercetin and vitamin C, it also contains lycopene, which has linked significance to lower blood pressure. Just do not try to get a tomato from bottled tomato sauce of ketchup because it has a combination of salt and sugar in most recipes, resulting in increased blood sugar and blood pressure levels.

21. **Lima beans**: It may not be a tempting option for kids, but it has an excellent benefit for people who wants to lower down their blood pressure level because of its anti-inflammatory content. It is excellent for losing weight, too.

22. **Sweet potato**: Sweet potato not only helps you reduce blood pressure but also helps you lose weight. It contains high hypertension-fighting resistant starch and vitamin C, and beta-carotene. You may enjoy an oven-baked sweet potato fries for snacks.

23. **Broccoli**: One cup of broccoli provides 14% potassium, 8% magnesium, and 6% calcium needed for reduced blood pressure level. It is a popular source of a phytonutrient called glucosinolates, which

helps fight cancer. You may substitute many cooked entrees and side dishes with frozen broccoli.

24. **Fat-free plain yogurt**: One cup of fat-free plain yogurt contains 12% magnesium, 18% potassium, and 49% calcium that you need for a daily dose to reduce blood pressure. Cool and creamy yogurt is an excellent ingredient in mineral-rich breakfasts, in salad dressings and sauces, and even in entrees. There are yogurts, which are high in calcium content, but no matter what type you buy, make sure to stick to low-sugar and free of flavorings varieties.

25. **Bell pepper**: One cup of raw bell pepper contains 9% potassium, 4% magnesium, and 1% calcium that you need for a daily dose of blood pressure-lowering diet. You may keep red bell peppers in the refrigerator for up to 10 days. One tip is to store them wrapped in a slightly damp paper towel to prevent them from drying out. You can freeze extras to use later in cooked dishes.

26. **Hibiscus tea**: Drinking three servings of hibiscus tea every day for six weeks provides a significant effect in lowering blood pressure level, as it is filled with a high level of anti-oxidants. You may drink one in the morning, during snacks, and before sleeping, or when you are working.

27. **Avocado:** Half avocado contains 10% potassium, 5% magnesium, and 1% calcium, which are all necessary for a reduced blood pressure level. Aside from heart-healthy monounsaturated fats and pressure-soothing minerals, it also has health-promoting carotenoids. Even the dark green flesh just under the crisp skin of avocado has large amounts of these disease-fighting compounds. Make it out of smoothie or plain during snacks.

28. **Quinoa:** Cooked quinoa contains 15% magnesium, 4.5% potassium, and 1.5% calcium. This high-protein whole grain has a nutty, mild flavor, which contains many health-improving phytonutrients aside from a great amount of magnesium. You can cook it half the time it takes to make brown rice. Besides, it is gluten-free, so it also makes a great option if you have celiac disease or you are gluten intolerant. The largely available options of quinoa are the golden beige color, but black and red options are also available and worth a try for your blood pressure reduction diet.

29. **Beet**: Drinking beet juice helps reduce blood pressure levels both in short and long terms. Drink 250 milliliters (about 1 cup) of beet juice every day for four weeks for a significant effect. You can also add beats to your favorite salads, or prepare the vegetables as a healthful side dish.

30. **Fermented food**: Fermented foods are rich in probiotics, which is a helpful bacteria that play an essential role in maintaining gut health. Eating probiotics provide a modest effect on high blood pressure. For more enhanced results on maintaining healthy blood pressure, consume probiotics regularly for more than eight weeks and multiple species of

probiotic bacteria. Some of the useful fermented food to eat are miso, apple cider vinegar, kimchi, natural yogurt, tempeh, and kombucha.

A healthy diet and lifestyle are of great help in reducing the risk of high blood pressure. Incorporate these into a balanced diet and engaging in adequate physical activity can control blood pressure and improve overall health.

CHAPTER 4: WHAT NOT TO EAT WHEN YOU HAVE HIGH BLOOD PRESSURE

You must be aware of the foods that affect your blood pressure level negatively. There are many activities involving drinking and eating with family and friends, that can influence bad nutritional choices. It is therefore important to know and understand which foods to avoid.

1. **Alcohol:** Drinking alcohol can reduce heart disease risks, but only when consumed in recommended amounts and moderation. Drinking too much alcohol may result in long-term weight gain and initial dehydration, in which both have a consequent effect on the increased blood pressure level.

2. **Coffee:** Drinks that contain caffeine such as coffee may cause an essential increase in your blood pressure level, and it is terrible for the heart. Also, it may cause decreased libido. Caffeinated drinks cause the adrenal glands to release excess adrenaline and cortisol substances that commonly cause another increase in blood pressure.

3. **Soft drinks:** Soft drinks are filled with calories and sugar. One 12-oz soft drink contains 39 grams of sugar or equivalent to nine teaspoons of pure sugar. That amount is the recommended amount of sugar

intake for men, but that is for the entire everyday amount that must be taken in. On the other hand, women only need 2/3 of the total amount indicated, so it means that it already exceeded the maximum sugar intake that is recommended daily.

4. **Canned soup:** Canned soup is easy to prepare, particularly when you are not feeling well or when you are in a hurry. But canned soups contain high sodium, and the ingredients inside, such as stokes and broths, can be bad for the blood pressure level. There are evens soups, which have more or less 900mg of sodium in every one-half cup. It means that if you eat the whole can of soup, it is more than 2000 mg of sodium that you are taking. The best option is to go for reduced and/or low-sodium soups, or you can make your soup with a low-sodium recipe to keep the salt in check.

5. **Salt:** Salt is among the most problematic ingredients for those who have high blood pressure. While it is difficult to avoid, it is advisable not to have much intake of it. We all love to add salt in our food because it is the easiest way to modify or improve the flavor profile of any dish. It can also be challenging to tell if your food has lots of salt in it. If it is hard to cut the salt in your dishes, you can just focus on the other ingredients that have a more significant impact on making your dish taste better.

6. **Sugar:** Excessive intake of sugar has been linked to many cases of weight gain and obesity. Not only that, but sugar is also related to high blood pressure. Sugar and all other sugar-sweetened food and drink have a vital impact when it comes to obesity for people of all

ages. Thereby, increase blood pressure level is more common in people who are obese and/or overweight.

7. **Sauces and condiments:** When you were advised to cut on salt intake, you are more likely to use other condiments instead, such as soy sauce, salad dressings, steak sauce, and/or barbeque sauce. However, if you would look at the ingredients of sauces and condiments, you will see that they have lots of salt in them. Even white and red sauces in some Italian dishes have lots of salt, and this also includes gravy. On the other hand, to avoid these hidden salts, you may use spice blends that don't use salt instead. These include using cinnamon, basil, and ginger for bread, snacks, salads, or vegetables. You may also use chili powder, dill seed and weed, parsley, and rosemary for fish and meats; thyme, sage, and marjoram for chicken.

8. **Candy:** Candy has lots of sugar and calorie content, increasing your sugar levels tremendously. Avoid those candy bars and other sugary suckers. Instead, go for fruits that are naturally sweetened as they are also rich in potassium and fiber – important content for preventing and reducing blood pressure levels.

9. **Cheese:** Cheese contains lots of salt. A typical cheese contains more or less 500 mg of sodium per serving. Thereby, the next time you decide on which cheese to purchase, keep those numbers in mind and choose a lower-sodium option, choose a fresh mozzarella at 175 mg of sodium per ounce or Swiss cheese at less than 60 mg per ounce.

10. **Whole milk:** Milk is a good source of calcium, but whole milk has a high content of fat dairy, which provides more fat than what you need. One cup

serving of whole milk contains more or less 8 grams fat, with saturated ones of about 5 grams. In this case, saturated fats are worse as compared to other types of fats, and is associated with heart disease. For an alternative, you may take skim or try using 1 or 2% milk only.

11. **Frozen pot pies:** A single serving of pot pie contains more or less 1400mg sodium plus it contains 35g fat. In line with this, you are already taking 50% more of your recommended amount per day for both, and in just one serving. The fat in frozen pot pies also include trans fat, and this needs to be removed from your diet. You have to say no to pre-packed frozen meals from now on.

12. **Bacon:** Bacon is mostly fat, and three slices of it make 4.5 grams of fat already, along with 300mg of sodium. It is generally taken during breakfast, but people usually take more than three slices of bacon. Bacon in sandwiches is also more than three slices. It might be challenging to be a meat lover nowadays, but it is essential to go to healthy choices instead.

13. **Red meat:** One serving of a Texas-sized steak contains more than a thousand calories already and remember that fatty foods are bad for both the blood vessels and the heart. It even contains 1500mg sodium and 80g fat. You can still go for red meat, but make sure to make a healthy eating plan with a small amount so you can check the recommended amount to take.

14. **Deli meat:** Processed lunch and deli meats for the sandwich are a trap for excessive sodium intake. It is because deli meat is already seasoned, cured, and preserved with salt so that it would last longer. A 2-ounce service of the sandwich with deli meat for lunch could provide more or less 600mg of sodium. Aside from that, with additional cheese, bread, pickles, and some condiments, a simple sandwich is not a good option anymore.

15. **Baked goods:** Baked foods frequently come with sprinkles and colorful icing, which are very enticing, but these ingredients are filled with sugar, salted saturated fats, and even sodium. Overeating of baked foods like cookies, pastries, and cakes may lead to unhealthy weight gain and obesity, resulting in having a blood pressure problem in the future.

16. **Donut:** The donuts that you love are one of the number one food that must be avoided when you have high blood pressure. This snack is worse as compared to many other snacks that you can eat, because of the 54% carbs and 42% fat that it contains, plus more or less 300 calories for each ring-shaped dough. Furthermore, since the process of cooking donuts is through frying, it also contains trans and saturated fats, and these are more trans fat than

chocolate bars and peanut butter. Avoiding donuts is also healthier for your heart.

17. **Pickles:** This low-calorie snack is an excellent partner to your salad and sandwich, but it is not recommended for people with diabetes because it is filled with sodium. Three medium pickles may contain more or less 2500mg sodium, which is more than the advisable sodium intake of 2300mg for the whole day.

18. **Cup noodles:** Cup noodles and other pre-packed noodle meals are popular choices among college students and other lazy adults. However, this instant meal choice is not suitable for the body. One pack of generic ramen noodles provide the body with about 1600mg sodium and 15g fat.

19. **Frozen pizza:** It is another easy and affordable dinner option for most people. However, frozen pizzas are highly damaging to the body because of the sodium content that it provides. The combination of cured meat, crust, cheese, and tomato sauce adds up the amount of sodium very quickly. The worse thing is that it has lots of salt to preserve all that flavor in the freezer. One service of this food may have as much as a thousand milligrams sodium.

20. **Chinese takeout food:** Most Chinese food items have sodium content worth the two days of intake. For example, beef with broccoli is filled with 3000mg salt plus the ingredients from cooking the dish (such as teriyaki sauce and/or soy sauce) is filled with around 1000mg salt in just one tablespoonful. The oil used for tossing around the broccoli and beef also adds to the amount. It is the reason why even Chinese sauteed vegetables look very shiny.

If you discovered that you have high blood pressure, avoiding these food options can help you prevent or lower your blood pressure level. Eating with your high blood pressure in mind doesn't mean that you are depriving yourself. It is about eating smart and making healthy choices for your body.

CHAPTER 5: HIGH BLOOD PRESSURE SOLUTION VS. WEIGHT LOSS – WHAT'S THE DIFFERENCE?

Healthy eating and the right diet plan are the best solutions for prevention and control from health problems like diabetes, heart disease, some types of cancer, and high blood pressure. However, is the weight loss diet and high blood pressure solution diet the same? Well, they are correlated with each other because overweight is a risk factor for diabetes. The difference is that a weight loss diet can be used or helps reduce the blood pressure level, but not all high blood pressure solution diet foods are necessary for weight loss. You can lessen or prevent your risk of high blood pressure through weight loss. Even the small amounts of weight loss can make a huge difference in treating high blood pressure.

The calories in your food and drink provide the needed amount of energy for the body, but if you take in more calories than the maximum amount that your body needs, it is going to store those excess energies as fat. On the other hand, if you take fewer calories than what is needed for the body, it will burn the fat stored by your body to make up the difference. The best way to lose weight to an average level is by making small changes to your eating habits, along with the activities that you can keep. The easiest way of weight loss is through fewer calorie intake, as it takes a lot of effort to burn the same number of calories through other activities.

For instance, you usually drink a large latte with a chocolate stick or whole milk; it contains 220 calories, and neither of which takes longer to drink or eat. However, you need to walk more than one hour or do some cyclings for 50 minutes to burn that 220 calories. Eating food or drinks with too many fats or lots of added sugar can result in gaining weight and can make it more challenging to lose weight. By making healthier options, there is no need to eat less. You can also swap other foods with healthier ones, and it will make a real difference in having a healthy weight, and thus, healthy blood pressure. There are high-sugar drinks, and you can swap it with water or other sugar-free versions to save on unnecessary calories.

Maximize Protein

Protein is the essential nutrient for losing weight and for a better-looking body. Taking foods with high protein reduces appetite, improves metabolism, and changes the weight-regulating hormones. A good baseline for those who are also doing exercise moderately is taking around ½ to ¾ grams of protein per pound of bodyweight. For instance, if you weigh 70 kg, your diet to lose weight is to take just 90 to 150 grams of protein per day. It is helpful and practical for not only losing fat but also for losing muscle.

In a 30-gram protein, you can take 7 ounces of plain Greek yogurt, ¾ cup of cottage cheese, and 3 oz of turkey, lean beef, fish, or turkey. You can also get the protein of high quality from vegetables and some other plant-based foods like nuts, whole grains, tofu, and legumes. These are all vetter options as compared to eating processed meats. Include protein in every meal because it also helps you to feel fuller in a more extended period. But select proteins that do not contain high fat. Some examples of low-fat, high protein foods are fish, white meat without skin, and eggs.

Choose Fiber

Fiber is another weight loss nutrient that is usually being overlooked. A diet high in fiber has several benefits in losing weight, and thereby, a significant contributor to lowering the blood pressure level. While it is a carbohydrate, it cannot be digested easily; this means that it adds bulk to make you feel fuller after the meal while not boosting your calories or blood sugar. You will be able to eat and enjoy a more significant portion of foods with high fiber content and still keep your calories under control.

This nutrient comes only from plants, so make sure to include plant-based foods in your diet. The good thing about it is that these types of food sources also contain other nutrients like antioxidants, phytonutrients, and vitamins that can improve your health. Fiber is mainly found in seeds, plant membranes, and skin. Juices usually have little fiber content, and peeling the fiber-rich food will discard the valuable fiber nutrient.

Blackberries or raspberries has 8 grams of fiber, which makes it the most fiber-dense food to eat for losing weight. You can snack on them or add them to your yogurt bowl.

Other fruits with high-fiber content include guavas, pomegranate seeds, and passionfruit. Another great fiber additions are dried fruits like dates, figs, and raisins, but consider the portions because while these fruits are high in fiber content, they are also filled with sugar.

Colored vegetables are also high in fiber, and they are great satisfactory foods without providing that much calorie count. Examples are beets, brussels sprouts, parsnips, and carrots. You may also include vegetables like spinach, green peppers, and onions in your breakfast when you cook eggs.

Limit the serving portion

While you already know the significant food nutrients to take in losing weight (to result in lower blood pressure), you need to know how much you are going to eat. Even if you are eating healthy foods or the right foods, if you overeat, you are still putting on weight.

To control your portions, it is advisable to take your time over a meal. You will know when you have eaten enough and when to stop before you feel uncomfortably full. When cooking, weight your rice and pasta and stick to the recommended servings. Another helpful tip is to use smaller plates and bowls, and just add a side salad and vegetables to your plate so that it would not look empty.

Be realistic

Set a realistic goal for yourself when losing weight. You can just goal to lose around 5 to 10 percent of your total weight in a span of 3 to 6 mos. It is already good progress if you would be able to lose weight of around 0.5 to 1kg per week. There is no need to reach your ideal BMI weight to see progress and results. Achieving the ideal BMI is definitely great, but it put pressure on you, and it still provides excellent benefits when you can lose 5-10 percent of your overall weight.

Write down the food you are eating, when you eat and why. Note the nutrient intake that you have for a particular food. You can also note if you skip breakfast but ate a large portion of lunch. Writing these things down is like you are keeping a food diary, and it is helpful for you to set goals for yourself.

Choose whole-wheat over processed starches

People eating whole wheat will have improved resting metabolic rate and higher losses of feces as compared to those eating processed carbohydrates. Eating whole grains with the same amount of fiber intake helps you lose more or less an additional hundred calories every day than those who consume processed carbohydrates.

The extra calories that you lose from eating whole wheat are equivalent to a 30-minute walk. It means that you will be able to enjoy a new small cookie per day. On the other hand, you have to avoid starchy foods with predominantly white color, such as potatoes, rice, white bread, or pasta. Plus, whole wheat provides higher nutritional value and makes you much fuller (helpful in preventing you from overeating)

CHAPTER 6: EFFECTIVE MEAL PLAN TO HELP YOU REDUCE AND CONTROL HIGH BLOOD PRESSURE

This meal plan is specially made to help make life easier while learning what to and not to eat with high blood pressure. It is made simple to follow for busy people and to cook many servings, as long as you prepare in advance. The recipes are not too complicated, so it is very realistic for people who don't know much about cooking.

Day 1

Breakfast: 1 banana, one bowl of oats with milk

Lunch: Summer salad with balsamic vinaigrette

> ***Ingredients:***
>
> For the salad
>
> - Hard-boiled eggs (2)
> - Ear of corn (1)
> - Halved cherry tomatoes (1/2 cup)
> - Arugula (3 cups)

- Fresh mozzarella cheese or cheese curds (2 oz)

For the dressing

- Minced garlic (1 clove)
- Olive oil (3 tablespoons)
- Balsamic vinegar (2 tablespoons)
- Pepper and salt (to taste, just be mindful of the amount)

Instructions:

1. Steam the corn ear for five to seven mins. Cut off the kernels. Set aside.
2. Combine all the ingredients for the dressing and shake well.
3. Assemble each salad by adding 1 1/2 cups arugula to each bowl and adding 1/2 of each of the rest of the ingredients.

Dinner: Apple Pecan Chicken (less bacon)

Ingredients:

- Shredded apple, tightly packed (1/4 cup)
- Skinless, boneless chicken breasts (1 pound)
- Pecans, chopped (1/2 cup)
- Hummus (3 tablespoons)
- Diced bacon (1 strip) – optional

Instructions:

1. Preheat oven to 200 degrees Celsius.
2. Put the shredded apple in a paper bowl. Squeeze to remove the excess moisture.
3. Combine bacon, apple, and hummus in a small pan.
4. Pat chicken dry with a paper towel (or you may rub it lightly with flour to coat). Place on a baking sheet.
5. Spread the mixture of hummus on top of the chicken to coat.
6. Top with the pecans and press it lightly to the hummus to help them stick.
7. Bake at 200 degrees Celsius for 20 minutes or until the chicken is cooked through.

Snacks (anytime): A handful of roasted almonds or plain cashews.

Day 2:

Breakfast: Salsa and egg toast

Ingredients:

- Olive oil (1/4 teaspoon)
- Whole-wheat bread, toasted (1 slice)
- Egg (1, large)
- Salsa (2 tablespoons)
- Kosher salt and pepper
- Banana (1, medium)

Instructions:

1. Toast the whole wheat bread.
2. Cook the egg in olive oil, or you may coat the pan with a thin layer of cooking spray.
3. Season with a pinch each of salt and pepper.
4. Top toast with salsa and egg.
5. Add one medium banana to your breakfast.

Lunch: White beans and vegetable salad

Ingredients:

- White beans, rinsed (1/3 cup)
- Vegetables of your choice (3/4 cup) – you may try tomatoes and cucumber

- Mixed greens (2 cups)
- Diced avocado (1/2 cup)
- Olive oil (2 teaspoons)
- Red wine vinegar (1 tablespoon)
- Pepper, ground

- **Instructions:**
  1. Combine all ingredients.
  2. Then, top your salad with two teaspoons of olive oil, one tablespoon of red wine vinegar, and freshly ground pepper.

Dinner: Garlic Roasted Salmon and Brussels Sprouts / Cooked Lentils

Ingredients:

- Chopped fresh oregano, divided (2 tablespoons)
- Extra-virgin olive oil (1/4 cup)
- Garlic, divided (14 large cloves)
- Wild-caught salmon fillet skinned and cut into six portions (2 pounds)
- White wine, preferably Chardonnay (3/4 cup)
- Brussels sprouts, trimmed and sliced (6 cups)
- Lemon wedges
- Freshly ground pepper, divided (3/4 teaspoon)
- Salt, divided (1 teaspoon)

o **Instructions:**

1. Preheat oven to 230 degrees Celsius.
2. Mince two garlic cloves and combine with oil in a small bowl. Combine with ½ tbsp/ salt, 1 tbsp. Oregano, and ¼ tsp. Pepper.
3. Put 3 tbsp — seasoned oil in a large roasting pan.
4. Helve the remaining garlic cloves and toss with Brussels sprouts and add to the oiled pan. Roast for 15 minutes, stirring once.
5. Add wine to the remaining oil mixture. Remove the pan from the oven. Stir the vegetables and place salmon on top. Then, drizzle with wine mixture.
6. Sprinkle the remaining ½ tsp. of pepper and salt and 1 tbsp and oregano.
7. Bake until the salmon is just cooked through. Bake for 5-10 minutes more.
8. Serve with lemon wedges.

Add ½ cup of cooked lentils seasoned with a pinch of pepper and salt to your dinner.

Snacks (anytime): 1 medium orange or ¾ cup of blueberries

Day 3

Breakfast:

- Decaffeinated coffee
- Orange (1 medium)
- Fat-free milk (1 cup)
- Whole-wheat bagel (commercial) with 2 tbsp. peanut butter (no salt)

Lunch: Spinach salad

Ingredients:

- Sliced pear (1)
- Slivered almonds (1/3 cup)
- Fresh spinach leaves (4 cups)
- Canned mandarin orange sections (1/2 cup)
- Red wine vinaigrette (2 tablespoons)

Instructions:

1. Combine all ingredients in a bowl.

Add 1 cup of fat-free milk to your lunch, and you may eat 12 low-sodium wheat crackers.

Dinner:

- Brown rice pilaf with vegetables (1/2 cup)
- Fresh green beans, steamed (1/2 cup)

- Herb-crusted baked cod, 3 oz cooked (and around 4 oz raw)
- Fresh berries with chopped mint (1 cup)
- Herbal iced tea

Snacks (anytime): 4 vanilla wafers, 1 cup low-calorie fat-free yogurt

Day 4

Breakfast: Creamy coconut milk quinoa pudding

Ingredients:

- Uncooked quinoa (white, red, tri-color), drained and rinsed (3/4 cup)
- 100% pure maple syrup (2 tablespoons)
- Light coconut milk (1 can/14 ounce)
- Vanilla bean paste or vanilla extract (1 teaspoon)
- For garnishing: Fresh blueberries and whipped cream (1 tablespoon)

Instructions:

1. Bring quinoa and coconut milk in a small saucepan. Boil over high heat.
2. Lower the fire to medium-low and add in vanilla and maple syrup. Continue to cook for 30 minutes (stir occasionally) until the mixture is creamy and the pudding light consistency.
3. Place the mixture in a bowl in the refrigerator to cool down for several hours.
4. Serve around ½ to ¾ cup of pudding in a small dish.
5. Garnish with a handful of fresh blueberries and dollop of whipped cream.

6. Add one tablespoon walnuts or almond slices if you want, chopped.

You may swap maple syrup for honey if you do not have it.

Lunch: Choose your favorite/leftovers/eat out

Dinner: Bibimbap Nourishing Bowl

Ingredients:

- Brown rice (1/2 cup)
- Medium rainbow carrot, peeled and julienned (1)
- Swiss chard without stems or spinach, chopped (1 cup)
- Medium courgette, julienned (1)
- Eggs (2)
- Green onions, green parts only, chopped (1 handful)
- Extra-firm tofu (1/2 block)
- Water (1 cup)
- Olive oil (3 tablespoons)
- Pinch of salt
- Sesame seeds (optional)

Instructions:

1. Place rice in a saucepan with a pinch of salt and boiling water. Cook on low heat until all the water has been absorbed and rice is cooked.

2. Slice half of the tofu block into another half. Then, wrap with a paper towel. Place a plate and heavy object on top of the tofu. Set aside for 15mins. It helps tofu to drain faster. After pressing the tofu, cut it into medium rectangular

strips and coat both sides with salt. Grill the tofu in a hot grill pan for 5mins per side, or until it becomes golden brown or becomes crispy.

3. For the zucchini, spinach, and carrots, heat two tablespoons of olive oil in a skillet, then saute the vegetables (one at a time) with salt until they become tender. Zucchini will take about 2-4 minutes, spinach about 5-7 minutes, and carrots around 5 minutes.

4. Fry eggs with one tablespoon olive oil and a pinch of salt.

5. Place rice in 2 bowls, top with tofu and vegetables, and finish with a sunny side up egg.

6. Top it with sesame seeds (optional) and green onions. Stir everything up and serve.

Snacks (anytime): Sweet potato chips (It is recommended to soak the potato for one hour before cooking to remove some starch. It will make it crispy to bake).

Day 5

Breakfast: Choose your favorite

Lunch: Fresh spring (rice paper) rolls

Ingredients:

- Bell pepper, any color, sliced julienne style (1)
- Rice paper spring roll wrappers (12 pcs)
- Shredded romaine lettuce (2 cups)
- Cilantro, chopped (1 bunch)
- Carrots, peeled and sliced julienne style (2 large pieces)
- Avocado, sliced thin (1)
- Small cucumber and/or zucchini, sliced julienne style (1)
- Scallion, white, and green parts, chopped (1)
- Shredded red cabbage (1 cup)
- Sauce of your choice recommended is a Thai peanut sauce

- **Instructions:**

    1. Before starting, lightly wet your workspace so that you can prevent your rice paper wrapper from sticking.

    2. Take one dry rice spring roll wrapper and place it in the bowl of lukewarm water. Let the rice paper sit in the water for ten to twenty seconds, or until it becomes pliable.

    3. Continue to feel how flexible the rice paper is (this is the tricky part). You want it to be workable and soft without being mushy.

    4. When the rice paper is ready, take the wrapper out of the water and lay it down flat on your wet surface.

    5. Starting in the center of the wrapper, place the zucchini, carrot, and bell pepper in a rectangular shape, and have it far from the edges of the wrapper.

    6. Continue adding all of the fillings, from cilantro to the purple cabbage. Place everything in the center, one by one, but maintain the rectangle shape in the middle. It is essential to work fast to prevent the wrapper from falling apart. However, do not overfill the wrapper as it will again cause the wrapper to tear.

    7. Enjoy with your favorite dipping sauce, or you may try the Thai peanut sauce this time.

Dinner: Honey lime chicken kebabs

Ingredients:

- grated lime rind (2 tsp)
- Chili powder (1 tsp) - optional
- Boneless, skinless chicken breast – cut into 1-inch cubes (1 pound)
- Kosher salt (1/4 tsp)
- Honey (1 tbsp)
- Fresh lime juice (2 tbsp)
- Minced garlic (2 tsp)
- Cooking spray

Instructions:

1. Preheat the broiler high.
2. Combine the first five ingredients, toss to coat. Thread the chicken onto eight skewers, 6 inches.
3. Place the kebabs on a broiler pan coated with cooking spray. Broil for 4mins on each side or until it is done.
4. Combine honey and juice in a small bowl, stir with a whisk. Arrange kebabs on a platter, drizzle with honey mixture and sprinkle with chili powder (optional).

Snacks (anytime): Healthy microwave popcorn

Ingredients:

- Popcorn

Instructions:

1. Measure out around ¼ cups of popcorn kernels and pour them into a paper lunch bag.
2. Fold the top over a few times to close, and place in the microwave. Use the popcorn button and listen carefully. When you hear the pops are slowing down to several seconds between pops, take it out and enjoy your popcorn.
3. Season if you want, but do not go overboard.

Day 6

Breakfast: Chocolate peanut butter smoothie

Ingredients:

- Cocoa (3 tablespoons)
- Honey (1 tablespoon) – optional
- Peanut butter (2 tablespoons)
- Banana, cut into chunks and frozen (1)
- Plain Greek yogurt (3/4 cup)
- Milk (3/4 cup)

Instructions:

1. Place all ingredients in the blender.
2. Turn on low and slowly up to high speed.
3. Blend until it becomes smooth.

Lunch: Roasted sweet potato salad

Ingredients:

- Medium sweet potato, peeled and cut into 1-in. chunks (1)
- Yellow or red bell pepper, seeded and finely diced (1/2)
- Chopped red onion (a few tablespoons)
- Black beans (1 cup)

- Minced jalapeno (1/2)
- Minced garlic (1 clove)
- Zest of lime or lemon (1)
- Chopped fresh cilantro (1/3 cup)

Instructions:

1. Heat oven to 200 degrees Celsius. Put red peppers, jalapenos, sweet potatoes, and garlic on a large baking sheet.

2. Drizzle with olive oil, toss to coat, and spread out in one layer. Sprinkle with pepper and salt. Roast until the potatoes start to brown on corners and just tender, occasionally turn, for around 30-40 mins. After removing from oven, keep on pan until ready to be mixed with the other ingredients.

3. Combine lime/lemon zest, cilantro, red onion, and black beans in a small bowl. Add the sweet potato mixture and drizzle with a little more olive oil. Then, season with pepper and salt.

4. Serve warm or at room temperature. You can refrigerate it for up to one day.

Dinner: Leftovers/choose your favorite/eat out

Snacks (anytime): 1 banana

Day 7

Breakfast: Apple walnut quinoa

Ingredients:

- Quinoa uncooked (1 cup)
- Coconut oil or butter (2 tablespoons)
- Medium apple, thinly sliced (2 pcs)
- Water for quinoa (3 cups)
- Juice and zest of an orange (1 pc)
- Cinnamon (1/2 teaspoon)
- Walnuts (1/4 cup)
- Kosher salt (1/2 teaspoon)

Instructions:

1. Melt the coconut oil in a pot with medium heat.
2. Add slices of apple in one layer. Sprinkle with half of the amount of orange zest, and juice, and cinnamon.
3. Let the apple cook on medium-low heat until it starts caramelizing, around 10mins. Stir often to avoid burning.
4. Add dry quinoa when the apples are mostly caramelized. Then, toast for one minute.
5. Add salt and water, and the rest of the orange juice. Turn heat to high to boil.

6. Reduce to simmer and cook until the water is thoroughly absorbed. It would take around 15 minutes.

7. Then, toast the walnuts until fragrant on a separate bowl.

8. Garnish with walnut and the remaining orange zest.

Lunch: Pumpkin Soup

Ingredients:

- Pumpkin (500 grams)
- Whole onions, skin on (2)
- Salt and pepper
- Whole knob of garlic, skin on (1)

Instructions:

1. Chop the pumpkin skin off and cut the pumpkin into wedges. Cut them into rough pieces. The bigger the size, the longer it will take for them to be cooked.

2. Bake on a tray lined with non-stick baking paper at 180 degrees Celsius oven for around 30 to 40 minutes, or until the pumpkin becomes soft.

3. As you remove them, get a big saucepan ready on the stove to prepare the soup. Then, squeeze the onion out from their skins into the pan, same with the knob of garlic, and discard the skins. Place the pumpkin into the pan.

4. Add 1.5 liters vegetable or chicken stock, and let boil for 5 minutes.

5. Remove from heat and blend with a stick blender until it gets smooth. Serve.

Dinner: Walnut bolognese and green lentil served with any pasta.

Snacks (anytime): A handful of roasted almonds or plain cashews.

Day 8

Breakfast: Grapefruit green smoothie

Ingredients:

- Plain yogurt (1/2 cup)
- Grapefruit (1/2)
- Almond milk (3/4 cup)
- Ginger root, peeled (1 inch)
- Spinach (1 cup)
- Banana (1/2)

Instructions:

1. Cut the peel off of the grapefruit and slice into large pieces. Place into the blender with all other ingredients and puree until it becomes smooth.

Lunch: Quinoa salad with nuts

Ingredients:

- Quinoa, any colors (1/2 cup)
- Spring onions or small red onion, finely sliced and diced (4pcs)
- Kale, shredded (2 cups)
- Sesame seeds, toasted (1/4 cup)
- Pumpkin seeds, toasted (1/4 cup)
- Sunflower seeds, toasted (1/4 cup)

- Cashews, toasted and roughly chopped (1/4 cup)
- Almonds, toasted and roughly chopped (1/4 cup)
- Kale, shredded (2 cups)
- Small red capsicum, finely diced (1)
- Coriander, chopped (1/2 bunch)
- Mint, chopped (1/2 bunch)
- Medium carrots, grated (2 cups)
- Pomegranate seeds for garnishing - optional

For the dressing:

- Maple syrup or honey (2 tsp)
- Salt (1/4 to ½ tsp)
- Extra virgin olive oil (1/4 cup)
- Garlic, crushed (1 clove)
- Apple cider vinegar or freshly squeezed lemon juice (1/4 cup)

Instructions:

1. Cook quinoa in a saucepan and cover generously with cold water, then boil.
2. Turn the heat down and simmer for around 15 minutes, or until it becomes soft. Note: it will take approximately 20 minutes to cook if you are using black quinoa.

3. Drain well and set aside to cool for around 5 to 10 minutes.

4. Prepare all other herbs, nuts, vegetables, and seeds for the salad.

5. For the dressing, add lemon juice, garlic, salt, olive oil, and honey to a jar with a tight-fitting lid.

6. Shake well to combine the ingredients.

7. When quinoa is cooled slightly, add the dressing and stir through.

8. Add kale, herbs, capsicum, onions, and carrot. Stir to combine.

9. Add the nuts and seeds just before serving. Stir through.

10. Top with pomegranate seeds (optional)

Dinner: Healthy chipotle chicken sweet potato skins

Ingredients:

- Medium sweet potatoes (3)
- Skinless, boneless chicken breast (3/4 pound)
- Whole chipotle pepper, minced (3)
- Spinach (2 cups)
- Greek yogurt, for serving (1 tablespoon)
- Fresh lime juice (2 tablespoons)
- Olive oil (1/4 cup)
- Chili powder (2 teaspoons)
- Dried oregano (1 teaspoon)
- Sharp white cheddar cheese, grated (5 ounces)
- Cumin (1 teaspoon)
- Garlic, grated or minced (2 cloves)

Instructions:

1. Preheat oven to 180 degrees Celsius. Wash the sweet potatoes and prick all over with a fork. Place them in the oven to bake for around 50-60mins or until it becomes fork-tender.

2. Then, place the chicken in a baking dish. Rub with one tbsp olive oil, pepper, and salt. Place in the oven with potatoes and bake for around 25mins. Cool it down and shred the chicken using your hands or using a fork. When potatoes are cut in half, cool it for 5 to 10mins.

3. Meanwhile, combine the lime juice, chipotle peppers, olive oil, cumin, salt, pepper, chili powder, oregano, and garlic in a medium-size bowl. Set aside.

4. Wilt the spinach in a small skillet over medium heat fire. Toss the shredded chicken and the spinach together. Set aside and keep warm.

5. Turn the oven up to 200 degrees Celsius. Scrape the sweet potato out of the peel, and leave a medium-size layer of flesh inside, with the peels to stand up on its own — place in a baking dish.

6. Brush the potato skins with a little chipotle sauce. Bake for around 5 to 10mins or until it looks crisp and nice.

7. While baking, mix the chicken, chipotle sauce, and spinach. Remove the skins from oven and stuff with the chicken mixture. Then top it with shredded cheese. Bake again for another 10mins or just until the cheese melts and skins become crisp and hot.

8. Serve with Greek yogurt and fresh chopped cilantro if desired.

Snack (anytime): 5 to 7 ounces plain Greek yogurt and one small banana

Day 9

Breakfast: Healthy banana and chocolate-peanut butter smoothie bowl

Ingredients:

- Skim milk (1/4 cup)
- Frozen banana, diced (1)
- Cocoa powder (1 tablespoon)
- Rolled oats (1/4 cup)
- Vanilla (1/4 teaspoon)
- Honey, to taste (1 teaspoon)
- Plain Greek yogurt (1/2 cup)
- Natural peanut butter (1 tablespoon)
- Cocao nibs
- Sliced banana
- Crushed peanuts

Instructions:

1. Blend the yogurt, peanut butter, oats, milk, vanilla, honey, banana, and cocoa powder in a food processor or blender. Pour into a bowl.
2. Top it with cocoa nibs, bananas, and crushed peanuts.

Lunch: Canned tuna (in water or oil), and salad

Dinner: Crunchy Broccoli Salad

Ingredients:

- Fresh broccoli florets (around 1 lb, 8 cups)
- Dried cranberries (1/2 cup)
- Sunflower kernels (1/4 cup)
- Canola oil (3 tbsp)
- Cooked and crumbled bacon strips (3 strips)
- Thinly sliced green onion (1 bunch)
- Sugar (2 tbsp)
- Seasoned rice vinegar (3 tbsp)

Instructions:

1. In a large bowl, combine the cranberries, broccoli, and green onions. On the other hand, in a small bowl, whisk vinegar, sugar, and oil until blended.
2. Drizzle over the broccoli mixture and toss to coat.
3. Refrigerate until serving.
4. Sprinkle with bacon and sunflower kernels before serving.

Snack (anytime): cucumber sticks and carrot sticks (1 cup)

Day 10

Breakfast: Peanut-butter cinnamon toast. Spread toast with peanut butter, top with banana slices and sprinkle with cinnamon.

Lunch: Salmon pita sandwich

Ingredients:

- Nonfat yogurt (2 tbsp)
- Lemon juice (2 tsp)
- Whole-wheat pita bread (1/2, 6 inches in size)
- Fresh dill, chopped (2 tsp)
- Canned sockeye salmon, flaked and drained (3 oz)
- Prepared horseradish (1/2 tsp)
- Watercress (1/2 cup)

Instructions:

1. Mix lemon juice, horseradish, dill, and yogurt in a bowl. Stir in salmon.
2. Stuff the pita half with the watercress and salmon salad.

Dinner: Quinoa Tabbouleh

Ingredients:

- Rinsed quinoa (1 cup)

- Minced fresh parsley (1/3 cup)
- Peeled and chopped cucumber (1 pc, small)
- Black beans, rinsed and drained (1 can, 15 oz)
- Water (2 cups)
- Pepper (1/2 tsp)
- Salt (1/2 tsp)
- Lemon juice (1/4 cup)
- Olive oil (2 tbsp)

Instructions:

1. Boil water in a large saucepan. Add quinoa. Lower the heat, cover, and simmer it for around 12 to 15mins or until the liquid is completely absorbed. Remove from heat and fluff with a fork. Transfer to a bowl and cool.

Add the red pepper, cucumber, beans, and parsley. In a small bowl, whisk the remaining ingredients and drizzle over salad. Toss to coat.

Snacks (anytime): 1 cup raspberries or cinnamon pears (sprinkle cinnamon to pear slices)

Day 11

Breakfast: Yogurt with raspberries and nuts. Top yogurt with walnut, raspberries, and honey

Lunch: White Bean Avocado Toast

Ingredients:

- Avocado, mashed (1/4)
- Whole wheat bread, toasted (1 slice)
- Kosher salt
- Ground pepper
- Red pepper, crushed (optional)
- Canned white beans, rinsed and drained (1/2 cup)

Instructions:

1. Top whole-wheat toast with white beans and mashed avocado.
2. Season with a pinch of pepper, salt, and crushed red pepper.

Add ½ cup of cucumber slices and 1 ½ cups of mixed greens to your lunch.

Dinner: Stuffed Sweet Potato with Hummus

Ingredients:

- Large sweet potato, scrubbed (1 pc)
- Canned black beans, rinsed (1 cup)

- Chopped kale (3/4 cup)
- Hummus (1/4 cup)
- Water (2 tbsp)

Instructions:

1. Prick sweet potato all over using a fork. Bake on a microwave on high heat until it is cooked through, around 8-10mins.

2. Meanwhile, wash the kale and drain. Allow the water to cling to the leaves. Then, place it in a saucepan. Cover and cook over medium-high heat. Make sure to stir at least once or twice or until it's wilted. Add the beans. Then add one or two tbsp of water if the pot is dry. Continue cooking and occasionally stir, until the mixture steams hot, or around 1-2mins.

3. Split the sweet potato open and top it with the bean and kale mix. Combine 2 tbsp water and hummus in a small dish. Add additional water if necessary, to reach the desired consistency. Then drizzle the hummus dressing over the stuffed sweet potato.

Snacks (anytime): 1 medium plum

Day 12

Breakfast: Oats Idli

Ingredients:

For fried mixture

- Carrot, finely chopped (1 cup)
- Coriander leaves, chopped (1/2 cup)
- Urad dal (1 teaspoon)
- Oil (1 tablespoon)
- Mustard seeds (1 teaspoon)
- Turmeric powder (1/2 teaspoon)
- Chana dal (1 teaspoon)
- Green chili (1 piece)
- Pinch of salt

For oats

- Oats (2 cups)

For idli batter

- Curd (2 cups)
- Salt (1 teaspoon)
- Pinch of fruit salt

Instructions:

For fried mixture

1. Heat oil over medium fire. Add the mustard seeds and let them crackle.

2. Add urad and chana dal, then the green chilis and turmeric powder. Mix them well and saute until they become light brown.

3. Then, add the coriander leaves and carrots (chopped finely). Combine all ingredients thoroughly and add a pinch of salt — Cook for 1-2 minutes.

4. Let it cool down for several minutes before you add it to the idli batter. Set aside.

For oats powder

1. Take the oats (2 cups) in a pan; dry roast for around 5mins or until it becomes golden brown.

2. Let it cool down. Grind it to make the oats powder.

For idli batter

1. Transfer the prepared oats powder to a big bowl. Add the fried mixture and a pinch of salt. Combine them well.

2. Add the necessary quantity of curd and stir thoroughly in one direction while adding a pinch of fruit salt.

3. Prepare a medium thick batter. Leave it covered for several minutes.

4. Grease the idli moulds with ghee with a brush.

5. Pour the oats idli batter in every mould. Then, put them in the steamer.
6. Cover with a lid — steam for around 15mins over medium fire.
7. Check if the idlis are cooked well after 15mins.

Lunch: Spicy Quinoa Crusted Chicken

Ingredients:
- Egg whites, beaten (2 pieces)
- Quinoa (1/2 cup)
- Shredded parmesan cheese (4 tbsp)
- Lime juice (1 tbsp)
- Water (1 cup)
- Cumin (1 tsp)
- Paprika (1/8 tsp)
- Black pepper (1/4 tsp)
- Chili powder (1 tsp)
- Salt (1/4 tsp)
- Cayenne pepper (1/4 tsp)
- 4 oz skinless, boneless chicken breasts (4 pcs)
- Optional: cilantro, light ranch dressing, lime wedges

Instructions:

1. Preheat oven at 150-degree Celsius and line a rimmed baking sheet with parchment paper. Set aside.

2. Heat a saucepan with high heat. Add one cup of water. Add the quinoa. Boil. After boiling, lower the fire to low. Cover and cook for around 8 to 10mins or until the quinoa is cooked.

3. Remove quinoa from heat and let stand for 5mins. Uncover. Stir in the salt, paprika, cumin, cayenne, chili powder, and pepper.

4. Evenly spread the cooked quinoa on the baking sheet and toast for 20 to 35mins, or until it dried out.

5. Allow the toasted quinoa to cool enough to handle, and have it transferred to a shallow dish or bowl.

6. Discard parchment paper; save the baking sheet. Line it with foil. Then, spray with nonstick cooking spray. Raise the oven heat to 180 degrees Celsius.

7. In a separate bowl, whisk the lime juice and egg white together.

8. Dip each chicken breast in the egg mixture and coat in the toasted quinoa. Press lightly to adhere to all sides.

9. Place the coated chicken breasts on the baking sheet. Place 1 tbsp of cheese on each, and bake for around 16 to 18mins.

10. Serve with a lime wedge, ranch dressing, and cilantro for garnish (optional).

Dinner: Your choice

Snacks: 1 cup raspberries

Day 13

Breakfast: Mediterranean Omelette

Ingredients:

- Eggs (3 pcs)
- Oregano (1 tbsp)
- White onion (2 tbsp)
- Olive oil (2 tbsp)
- Olives (2 tbsp)
- Spinach, blanched with butter (1 tbsp)
- Pepper and salt to taste

Instructions:

1. Whip the eggs lightly and add pepper and salt.
2. Heat oil in a pan and cook the whipped eggs.
3. Take a fork and stir the eggs gently.
4. Spread spinach, oregano, onions, and olives on top and fold.
5. Once done, fold it again.

Lunch: Oven-Baked Fried Green Tomatoes

Ingredients:

- Green tomatoes, around three large ones (1 ½ pound)

- Panko bread crumbs (1/2 cup)
- Low-fat parmesan cheese (1/4 cup)
- Low-fat buttermilk (1/3 cup)
- Ground flax meal (1/4 cup)
- Paprika (1/4 tsp)
- Cayenne pepper (1/2 tsp)
- Garlic powder (1/4 tsp)
- Onion powder (1/4 tsp)
- Hot sauce (1 tsp)
- Salt and pepper to taste

Instructions:

1. Preheat oven to 180 degrees Celsius and coat a baking sheet lightly with non-stick cooking spray. Set aside.
2. Slice tomatoes into 12 ¼ to ½ inch slices.
3. Set up two shallow bowls. Fill one with the hot sauce and buttermilk. In the other bowl, mix paprika, parmesan cheese, garlic powder, onion powder, flax, cayenne pepper, flax, pepper, and salt.
4. Dip each tomato slice in the buttermilk mixture, allowing the excess to drop off and transfer it to the panko mixture. Press the breadcrumbs lightly on the tomato on both sides.

5. Arrange the tomato slices in one layer on a baking sheet. Bake for around 25 to 30mins. Flip halfway through.

Dinner: Skinny Tilapia Lettuce Wraps

Ingredients:

- Diced tomatoes (2 cups)
- Tilapia fillets (2 lbs)
- Large romaine lettuce leaves (8 pcs)
- Diced onion (1 pc)
- Minced garlic (2 tbsp)
- Shredded red cabbage (1 cup)
- Fresh chopped cilantro (1/4 cup)
- Extra virgin olive oil (1 tsp)
- Lime juice (2 tbsp)
- Peeled and thinly sliced avocado (1 pc)
- Serrano pepper, seeded and diced (or jalapeno pepper) – 1 pc
- Salt (1/4 tsp)
- Black pepper to taste

Instructions

1. Heat a large skillet over medium fire. Add oil, serrano pepper, onions, and garlic. Cook for 2 to 4mins or until the onions start to soften.

2. Add fish to the skillet. Cook for 3 to 4mins on each side or until the fishes turn white and quickly flakes with a fork.

3. Turn heat to low fire. Break the tilapia up with a spatula or bend in the skillet. Add the lime juice, pepper and salt, cilantro, and tomatoes, and stir together gently — Cook for another 3 to 4mins.

4. Scoop 1/3 cup of tilapia mixture into each romaine leaf and top with the avocado slices and red cabbage evenly.

5. Each lettuce wrap is 4 oz of tilapia, ¼ of avocado, and 2 tbsp of red cabbage.

Snacks (anytime): 1 large Banana

Day 14

Breakfast: Spinach pancake

Ingredients:

Pancake

- Whole wheat flour (100g)
- Milk (100mL)
- Yogurt, whipped (150mL)
- Egg (1pc)
- Yolk (1pc)
- Vegetable oil (1tbsp)
- Water (3 tbsp)
- Pinch of nutmeg, grated
- Spinach leaves, drained, chopped to a paste, blanched (1/2 kg)

Dressing

- Salad/olive oil (3 tbsp)
- Pinch of sugar
- Pinch of mustard powder
- Salt and pepper
- Lemon juice (1 tbsp)
- Chopped garlic (1/2 tsp)

Filling

- Beaten hung curd (250 g)
- Grated cheese (100 g)
- Oil (1 tbsp)
- Egg (1 pc)
- Spring onions, sliced (3 tbsp)
- Sauteed mushrooms (250 g)
- Chopped parsley (2 tbsp)
- Pinch of chili powder
- Salt and pepper

Instructions:

Pancake

1. Sift flour into a bowl. Beat in egg, water, curd, and oil. Then, stir in the nutmeg, spinach pasta, and seasoning. Set aside for 30mins.

Dressing

1. Whisk the dressing ingredients together. Combine with herbs and seasoning, and tomatoes.

Filling

1. Heat oil and saute the onions for 2 to 3mins.

2. Beat onions into yogurt with the remaining ingredients, but use half of the cheese first.

3. Pour some batter into the oiled pan to form a thin pancake — Cook for around 2mins on each side.

4. Spread one tablespoon of filling over each pancake. Fold.

5. Arrange on an ovenproof buttered dish, scatter on remaining cheese and bake at 180-degree Celsius for 15mins.

6. Serve hot.

Lunch: Tomato Salad

Ingredients:

- Torn basil leaves (3 tbsp)
- Cherry tomatoes (1/2 kg)
- Salt and pepper

Instructions:

1. Mix cherry tomatoes and torn basil leaves. Add salt and pepper.

Dinner: Green Pea Upma

Ingredients:

Green pea Upma

- Semolina, roasted (1 cup)
- Finely chopped onion (1 pc)

- Green peas (1/4 cup)
- Green chilis, finely chopped (2 nos)
- Hot water (2 cups)

Tempering

- Curry leaves (1 sprig)
- Grated ginger (1 sprig)
- Mustard seeds (3/4 tsp)
- Extra virgin olive oil (1 tbsp)

Instructions:

1. Heat oil in a heavy-bottomed pan. Add the mustard seeds. Let it crackle.
2. Add grated ginger and curry leaves. Saute until ginger's raw aroma disappears.
3. Add finely chopped onion and saute until it becomes translucent. Now add the green chilis and saute for 2mins.
4. Add the semolina, lightly roasted. Add the green peas. Saute for 2mins and add the hot water after.
5. Add salt to taste. Then, stir to prevent lump formation.
6. Cover and cook on very slow fame. Cook until the water is absorbed, and the green peas and semolina are cooked.

Snacks (anytime): 1 cup cucumber

Day 15

Breakfast: Almond-banana porridge

Ingredients:

- Oats (1/4 cup)
- Milk (1 cup)
- Banana, chopped (1/2)
- Dates, chopped (1 tablespoon)
- Honey (1 tablespoon)
- Chia seeds (1 teaspoon)
- Sliced almonds (2 teaspoons)
- Cinnamon powder (2 teaspoons)
- Saffron thread (1 pc)

Instructions:

1. Soak oats in water for several minutes; soak chia seeds in another bowl with water for 10 mins.
2. Heat pan over medium fire and put milk. Add dates, cinnamon, banana, and almonds.
3. Add the saffron thread to milk. Add the oats after 30 seconds — Cook with the milk for 1 minute.
4. When the oats are cooked through, and the oatmeal (porridge) is in the right consistency,

remove the pan from fire and pour the porridge into a serving bowl.

5. Stir honey through the oatmeal porridge and garnish with chia seeds.

Lunch: Kale and Bean soup

Ingredients:

- Peeled and cubed potatoes (2 cups)
- Chopped onions (2 pcs, medium)
- Trimmed and coarsely chopped kale (1 bunch)
- Olive oil (1 tbsp)
- Minced garlic (4 cloves)
- Italian seasoning (1 tsp)
- Cannellini beans, rinsed and drained (1 can, 15 oz)
- Water (1 ½ cups)
- Vegetable broth (3 ½ cups)
- Pepper (1/2 tsp)
- Diced tomatoes, undrained (1 can, 12 oz)
- Paprika (1 tsp)
- Bay leaf (1 pc)

Instructions:

1. In a Dutch oven, saute potatoes and onions in oil until they become tender. Add garlic and cook for another minute.

2. Stir in the broth, water, paprika, bay leaf, kale, Italian seasoning, tomatoes, and pepper and let them boil. Lower the heat. Cover and simmer for 50 to 60 mins or until the kale becomes tender.

3. Cool slightly. Discard the bay leaf. Now in a blender, process 3 cups of soup until it becomes smooth. Return to pan and add beans. Then, heat through.

Dinner: Crunchy Broccoli Salad

Ingredients:

- Fresh broccoli florets (around 1 lb, 8 cups)
- Dried cranberries (1/2 cup)
- Sunflower kernels (1/4 cup)
- Canola oil (3 tbsp)
- Cooked and crumbled bacon strips (3 strips)
- Thinly sliced green onion (1 bunch)
- Sugar (2 tbsp)
- Seasoned rice vinegar (3 tbsp)

Instructions:

5. In a large bowl, combine the cranberries, broccoli, and green onions. On the other hand, in

a small bowl, whisk vinegar, sugar, and oil until blended.

6. Drizzle over the broccoli mixture and toss to coat.
7. Refrigerate until serving.
8. Sprinkle with bacon and sunflower kernels before serving.

Snacks (anytime): Greek yogurt

Day 16

Breakfast: Banana berry cereal (1 cup plain shredded wheat cereal with ½ cup of fat-free milk. Add one sliced medium banana and ½ cup blueberries)

Lunch: Spinach n Broccoli Enchiladas

Ingredients:

- Olive oil (2 tsp)
- 1% cottage cheese (1 cup)
- Chopped onion (1 pc, medium)
- Garlic powder (1/2 tsp)
- Flour Tortillas - warmed (8 pcs, 8 inches)
- Picante sauce, divided (1 cup)
- Frozen chopped spinach, thawed and squeezed dry (1 package, 10 oz)
- Ground cumin (1/2 tsp)
- Shredded low-fat cheddar cheese, divided (1 cup)
- Finely chopped fresh broccoli (1 cup)

Instructions:

1. Preheat oven to 350 degrees. In a large non-stick skillet, cook and stir onion in oil until tender, over medium fire. Add broccoli, spinach, garlic powder, 1/3 cup Picante sauce, and cumin. Heat the ingredients through.

2. Remove from fire. Stir in ½ cup cheddar cheese and cottage cheese. Spoon about 1/3 cup of spinach mixture down the center of each tortilla. Roll up and place seam side down in a baking dish that has a cooking spray. Spoon the remaining Picante sauce over the top.

3. Cover and bake for 20 to 25mins or until they are heated thoroughly. Uncover and sprinkle with the remaining cheese. Bake 5 mins more or until the cheese is melted.

Dinner: Apple Pecan Chicken (less bacon)

Ingredients:

- Shredded apple, tightly packed (1/4 cup)
- Skinless, boneless chicken breasts (1 pound)
- Pecans, chopped (1/2 cup)
- Hummus (3 tablespoons)
- Diced bacon (1 strip) – optional

Instructions:

1. Preheat oven to 200 degrees Celsius.
2. Put the shredded apple in a paper bowl. Squeeze to remove the excess moisture.
3. Combine bacon, apple, and hummus in a small pan.
4. Pat chicken dry with a paper towel (or you may rub it lightly with flour to coat). Place on a baking sheet.
5. Spread the mixture of hummus on top of the chicken to coat.
6. Top with the pecans and press it lightly to the hummus to help them stick.
7. Bake at 200 degrees Celsius for 20 minutes or until the chicken is cooked through.

Snacks: A handful of plain cashews

Day 17

Breakfast: Yogurt breakfast drink

Ingredients:

- Ice cubes (2 cups)
- Vanilla yogurt (2 cups)
- Peach yogurt (2 cups)
- Fat-free milk (1/2 cup)
- Thawed orange juice concentrate (1/2 cup)

Instructions:

1. In a blender, combine all ingredients except ice cubes. Cover; process until they become smooth. Add ice cubes, cover, and process again until smooth.

Lunch: Your choice/favorite

Dinner: Colorful quinoa salad

Ingredients

Salad

- Rinsed quinoa (1 cup)
- Grape tomatoes - halved (1 cup)
- Chopped green onions (2 pcs)

- Cucumber, seeded and chopped (1 pc, medium)
- Fresh baby spinach, thinly sliced (2 cups)
- Water (2 cups)
- Sweet yellow pepper, chopped (1 pc, medium)
- Sweet orange pepper, chopped (1 pc, medium)

Dressing

- Olive oil (2 tbsp)
- grated lime zest (1 tbsp)
- Lime juice (3 tbsp)
- Honey (4 tsp)
- Minced fresh ginger root (2 tsp)

Instructions:

1. Boil water in a large saucepan. Add quinoa. Lower the heat, simmer, and cover, until the liquid is completely absorbed, which might be around 12 to 15mins. Remove from heat, fluff with fork and transfer to a large bowl. Cool completely.

2. Stir the cucumber, green onions, spinach, peppers, and tomatoes into quinoa. In a small bowl, whisk dressing ingredients until they are blended well. Drizzle over quinoa mixture. Toss to coat and refrigerate until serving.

Snacks (anytime): Apple slices

Day 18

Breakfast: Bagel sandwich (3 oz whole wheat Bagel with one egg. Fried egg in a non-stick pan with cooking spray. Add ½ slice low-sodium Swiss cheese.

Lunch: Pistachio baked salmon

Ingredients:

- Pistachios, chopped (1 cup)
- Salmon fillets (6 pcs, 6 oz each)
- Lemon juice (3 tbsp)
- Pepper (1 tsp)
- Dill weed (1 tsp)
- Packaged brown sugar (1/2 cup)

Instructions:

1. Preheat oven to 220 degrees Celsius and place salmon in a greased baking dish. Combine the remaining ingredients and spoon over salmon.
2. Bake uncovered for around 12 to 15mins or until the fish easily flakes with a fork.

Dinner: Quinoa Tabbouleh

Ingredients:

- Rinsed quinoa (1 cup)
- Minced fresh parsley (1/3 cup)
- Peeled and chopped cucumber (1 pc, small)

- Black beans, rinsed and drained (1 can, 15 oz)
- Water (2 cups)
- Pepper (1/2 tsp)
- Salt (1/2 tsp)
- Lemon juice (1/4 cup)
- Olive oil (2 tbsp)

Instructions:

2. Boil water in a large saucepan. Add quinoa. Lower the heat, cover, and simmer it for around 12 to 15mins or until the liquid is completely absorbed. Remove from heat and fluff with a fork. Transfer to a bowl, and let it cool.

3. Add the red pepper, cucumber, beans, and parsley. In a small bowl, whisk the remaining ingredients and drizzle over salad. Toss to coat.

Snacks (anytime): 5 celery sticks filled with 1 tsp almond butter

Day 19

Breakfast: Ginger-kale smoothie

Ingredients:

- Torn fresh kale (2 cups)
- Lemon juice (1 tsp)
- Orange juice (1 ¼ cups)
- Minced fresh ginger root (1 tbsp)
- Apple, peeled and coarsely chopped (1 pc, medium)
- Dash cayenne pepper
- Ground cinnamon (1/8 tsp)
- Ice (4 cubes)
- Ground turmeric (1/8 tsp)

Instructions:

1. Place all ingredients in a blender and process until blended.

Lunch: Garlic Tilapia with spicy kale

Ingredients:

- Kale, trimmed and coarsely chopped (1 bunch, around 16 cups)
- Olive oil, divided (3 tbsp)
- Garlic salt (1/2 tsp)

- Fennel seed (1 tsp)
- Cannellini beans, rinsed and drained (1 can, 15 oz)
- Water (2/3 cup)
- Crushed red pepper flakes (1/2 tsp)
- Minced garlic (2 cloves)
- Tilapia fillets (4 pcs, 6 oz each)
- Pepper, divided (3/4 tsp)
- Salt (1/2 tsp)

Instructions:

1. Heat 1 tbsp oil over medium fire in a 6-qt stockpot. Add fennel, pepper flakes, and garlic. Cook and stir for 1 min. Add water and kale and boil. Simmer and cover for around 10 to 12mins or until the kale becomes tender.

2. In a separate bowl, sprinkle tilapia with ½ tsp garlic salt and pepper. In a large skillet, heat the remaining oil over medium flame. Add the tilapia and let it cook for 3 to 4mins on each side or until the fish starts to flake easily with a fork.

3. Add salt, beans, and the remaining pepper to kale. Heat through while stirring occasionally. Serve with tilapia.

Dinner: leftover/favorite

Snacks: Applesauce and graham crackers

Day 20

Breakfast: Melted milkshake (1 cup of fat-free milk mixed with 3 tbsp chocolate malt powder)

Lunch: Kale-fennel skillet

Ingredients:

- Fully cooked apple chicken sausage links or cooked Italian sausage links halved lengthwise and sliced into half-moons (1/2 lb)
- Dry white or dry sherry wine (3 tbsp)
- Extra virgin olive oil (2 tbsp)
- Pepper (1/8 tsp)
- Salt (1/8 tsp)
- Minced garlic (2 cloves)
- Fennel bulb, thinly sliced (1 pc, small)
- Onion, thinly sliced, (1 pc, small)
- Kale, trimmed and torn into bite-sized pcs (1 bunch)

Instructions:

1. Heat olive oil in a large skillet over medium-high fire. Add fennel and onion. Cook and stir for 6 to 8mins. Add garlic, seasonings, sausage, and sherry. Cook until the sausage begins to caramelize, or around 4 to 6mins.

2. Add kale, cook with a cover, but occasionally stirring, until the kale becomes tender. It might take 15 to 17mins.

Dinner: Berry nectarine salad

Ingredients:

- Nectarines, sliced (4 pcs, medium)
- Low-fat cream cheese (3 oz)
- Fresh blueberries (1 cup)
- Fresh raspberries (2 cups)
- Lemon juice (1 tsp)
- Sugar (1/4 cup)
- Ground ginger (1/2 tsp)

Instructions:

1. In a large bowl, toss nectarines with lemon juice, sugar, and ginger. Refrigerate with cover for around an hour and stir once.
2. Drain the nectarines but reserve the juices. Beat the reserved juices gradually into the cream cheese. Combine berries and nectaries gently. Serve with cream cheese mixture.

Snacks: Dried cherries

Day 21

Breakfast: Greek yogurt with ½ cup sliced strawberries and ¼ cup slivered almonds

Lunch: Easy glazed salmon

Ingredients:

- Unsweetened pineapple juice (1/4 cup)
- Packed brown sugar (1/3 cup)
- Salmon fillets (4 pcs, 6 oz each)
- Soy sauce (2 tbsp)

Instructions:

1. Line baking pan with foil and grease the foil. Set aside.
2. In a small bowl. Combine the pineapple juice, brown sugar, and soy sauce. Place salmon skin-side down on the prepared pan. Spoon the sauce mixture over the fish.
3. Bake without cover for 20 to 25 mins or until the fish flakes easily with a fork.

Dinner: Pumpkin Soup

Ingredients:

- Pumpkin (500 grams)
- Whole onions, skin on (2)
- Salt and pepper

- Whole knob of garlic, skin on (1)

Instructions:

6. Chop the pumpkin skin off and cut the pumpkin into wedges. Cut them into rough pieces. The bigger the size, the longer it will take for them to be cooked.

7. Bake on a tray lined with non-stick baking paper at 180 degrees Celsius oven for around 30 to 40 minutes, or until the pumpkin becomes soft.

8. Get a big saucepan ready on the stove to prepare the soup. Then, squeeze the onion out from their skins into the saucepan, same with the knob of garlic; discard the skins. Place the pumpkin into the saucepan.

9. Add 1.5 liters vegetable or chicken stock, and let boil for 5 minutes.

10. Remove from heat and blend with a stick blender until it gets smooth. Serve.

Day 22

Breakfast: Peanut butter toast (2 slices of low sodium whole wheat bread with 1 tbsp natural peanut butter

Lunch: Favorite/any of your choice.

Dinner: Skinny chickpea and vegetable pearl couscous

Ingredients:

- Diced zucchini (1 pc, large)
- Cumin (1 tsp)
- Water (1 ¼ cups)
- Extra virgin olive oil (3 tsp)
- Frozen peas, thawed (1 cup)
- Whole wheat pearl couscous (1 cup)
- Lemon juice (2 tbsp)
- Sliced scallions (3 pcs)
- Black pepper (1/4 tsp)
- Salt (1/2 tsp)
- Unsalted pistachios, chopped (3 tbsp)
- Diced tomato (1 pc, large)
- Chickpeas, drained and rinsed (1 pc, 15.5 oz)

Instructions:

1. In a medium saucepan, heat two teaspoons of olive oil over medium fire. Add zucchini and saute until it softens.

2. Stir in peas and scallions. Cook for another 2mins. Transfer to a bowl and cover with plastic wrap or foil to keep warm.

3. Mix the remaining teaspoons of olive oil with lemon, salt, pepper, cumin, and water in the same saucepan and boil. Stir in couscous, cover; turn heat to low. Let simmer for around 8 to 10mins. Make sure to stir occasionally.

4. Add the zucchini and chickpeas mixture. Let stand for 2mins. Sprinkle with pistachios and serve.

Day 23

Breakfast: Mediterranean Omelette

Ingredients:

- Eggs (3 pcs)
- Oregano (1 tbsp)
- White onion (2 tbsp)
- Olive oil (2 tbsp)
- Olives (2 tbsp)
- Spinach, blanched with butter (1 tbsp)
- Pepper and salt to taste

Instructions:

1. Whip the eggs gently and add pepper and salt.
2. Heat oil in a pan and cook the whipped eggs.
3. Take a fork and stir the eggs lightly.
4. Spread spinach, oregano, onions, and olives on top and fold.
5. Once done, fold it again.

Lunch: Healthy chipotle chicken sweet potato skins

Ingredients:

- Medium sweet potatoes (3)
- Skinless, boneless chicken breast (3/4 pound)

- Whole chipotle pepper, minced (3)
- Spinach (2 cups)
- Greek yogurt, for serving (1 tablespoon)
- Fresh lime juice (2 tablespoons)
- Olive oil (1/4 cup)
- Chili powder (2 teaspoons)
- Dried oregano (1 teaspoon)
- Sharp white cheddar cheese, grated (5 ounces)
- Cumin (1 teaspoon)
- Garlic, grated or minced (2 cloves)

Instructions:

1. Preheat oven to 180 degrees Celsius. Wash the sweet potatoes and prick all over with a fork. Place them in the oven to bake for around 50-60mins or until it becomes fork-tender.

2. Then, place the chicken in a baking dish. Rub with one tbsp olive oil, pepper, and salt. Place in the oven with potatoes and bake for around 25mins. Cool it down and shred the chicken using your hands or using a fork. When potatoes are cut in half, cool it for 5 to 10mins.

3. Meanwhile, combine the lime juice, chipotle peppers, olive oil, cumin, salt, pepper, chili

powder, oregano, and garlic in a medium-size bowl. Set aside.

4. Wilt the spinach in a small skillet over medium heat fire. Toss the shredded chicken and the spinach together. Set aside and keep warm.

5. Turn the oven up to 200 degrees Celsius. Scrape the sweet potato out of the peel; leave a medium size layer of flesh inside with the peels to stand up on its own — place in a baking dish.

6. Brush the potato skins with a little chipotle sauce. Bake for around 5 to 10mins or until it looks crisp.

7. While baking, mix the chicken, chipotle sauce, and spinach. Remove the skins from oven and stuff with the chicken mixture. Then top it with shredded cheese. Bake again for another 10mins or just until the cheese melts and skins become crisp and hot.

8. Serve with Greek yogurt and fresh chopped cilantro if desired.

Dinner: White Bean Avocado Toast

Ingredients:

- Avocado, mashed (1/4)
- Whole-wheat bread, toasted (1 slice)
- Kosher salt

- Ground pepper
- Red pepper, crushed (optional)
- Canned white beans, rinsed and drained (1/2 cup)

Instructions:

1. Top whole-wheat toast with white beans and mashed avocado.
2. Season with a pinch of pepper, salt, and crushed red pepper.

Add ½ cup of cucumber slices and 1 ½ cups of mixed greens to your dinner.

Day 24

Breakfast: Sweet potato toast with banana, almond butter, and toasted coconut chips

Ingredients:

- Banana, peeled and thinly sliced (1 pc, large)
- Sweet potatoes (2 pcs, medium, about 1 pound in total)
- Toasted coconut chips (1/4 cup)
- Almond butter (4 tablespoons)
- Coconut oil, melted (1 tablespoon)
- Fine salt

Instructions:

1. Preheat oven to 230 degrees Celsius.
2. Slice off the four long sides of each sweet potatoes to square off and sit flat on a cutting board. Then, slice them lengthwise into ½ inch thick planks, which would be around 5x2 inches. In a medium bowl, the sweet potatoes with a pinch of salt and the coconut oil and gently toss to coat. Spread them out on a baking sheet and roast (flip them halfway through until tender and browned. It may take around 15mins.
3. Divide the almond butter among the toasts and top each with sliced banana. Then, sprinkle them with toasted coconut.

Lunch: Red Curry with Vegetables

Ingredients:

- Lite coconut milk (1 can, 14 oz)
- Red Thai curry paste (1 to 2 tsp)
- Canola oil, divided (4 tsp)
- Fresh cilantro, chopped (1/3 cup)
- Extra-firm tofu, rinsed, patted dry and cut into 1-in cubes (1 package, 14 oz)
- Vegetable broth or low sodium chicken broth (1/2 cup)
- Brown sugar (1 tbsp)
- Green beans, trimmed and cut into 1-in pcs (1/2 lb)
- Sweet potato, cut into 1-in cubes (1 lb)
- Salt (1/2 tsp)
- Lime, quartered (1 pc)
- Lime juice (2 tsp)

Instructions:

1. In a large non-stick skillet, heat 2 tsp of oil over medium-high flame. Add tofu and cook. Make sure to stir it every 2-3 mins, or until it becomes brown, which may take 6-8 mins in total. Transfer to a plate.

2. Heat the remaining 2 tsp of oil over medium-high flame. Add the sweet potato and cook. Stir occasionally for 4-5mins or until it becomes

brown. Add broth, coconut milk, and curry paste. Boil.

3. Reduce to a simmer and cook with cover. Stir it occasionally for around 4mins or until the sweet potato is just tender. Add the green beans, tofu, and brown sugar. Return to a simmer and cook with cover. Stir occasionally until the green beans are tender-crisp, which is around 2-4mins. Stir in the salt and lime juice.

4. Sprinkle with cilantro. Serve with lime wedges.

Dinner: Creamy Gorgonzola Polenta with Summer Squash Saute

Ingredients:

- Crumbled Gorgonzola cheese (2/3 cup)
- Vegetable broth, or low-sodium chicken broth, divided (2 cans, 14 oz)
- Zucchini halved lengthwise and sliced (2 pcs, small)
- Fresh basil, chopped (1/4 cup)
- Extra virgin olive oil (2 tbsp)
- Cornmeal (3/4 cup)
- Yellow summer squash halved lengthwise and sliced (2 pcs, small)
- Water (1 cup)

- Minced garlic (3 tbsp)
- Flour (2 tbsp)
- Freshly ground pepper (1/2 tsp)

Instructions:

1. Mix 2 and ½ broth with one cup of water in a small saucepan. Boil. Then, whisk in pepper and cornmeal slowly until smooth. Reduce fire to low, cover and cook but make sure to occasionally stir until it becomes very thick and not grainy anymore, around 10-15mins. Stir in Gorgonzola. Remove from heat.

2. Meanwhile, in a large non-stick skillet, heat oil over medium-high fire. Add garlic and cook. Stir occasionally until it starts to soften and brown in places. Sprinkle the flour over the vegetables. Stir to coat.

3. Stir in the remaining one cup broth and boil. Stir it often. Then reduce fire to medium-low and simmer. Stir occasionally until it is thickened and the vegetables become tender. Stir in the basil. Serve the saute over the polenta.

Day 25

Breakfast: Crunchy pancakes

Ingredients:

- Granola (1/2 cup)
- Chia seeds (1 tablespoon)
- Flax seeds (1 tablespoon)
- Sunflower seeds (1 tablespoon)
- Brown sugar (2 tablespoons)
- Butter for frying
- Eggs (2 pcs, large)
- Whole grain pancake mix (2 cups)
- Vegetable oil (2 tablespoons)
- Milk (1 ½ cups)

Instructions:

1. Make the batter by mixing pancake mix, oil, milk, eggs, and brown sugar in a large bowl. Stir in the flax seeds, sunflower seeds, chia seeds, and granola.

2. Heat a non-stick skillet or griddle over medium heat and add a little butter. Drop-in around ¼ cup of batter each pancake and fry on both sides until it becomes dark golden. Continue with the remaining mixture. You may add more butter if needed.

Lunch: Lemony Lentil Salad with Salmon

Ingredients:

- Salmon, drained and flaked (2 cans, 7 oz), flaked cooked salmon (1 ½ cups)
- Lentils, rinsed (1 can, 15 oz) or cooked green or brown lentils (3 cups)
- Diced, seedless cucumber (1 cup)
- Lemon juice (1/3 cup)
- Extra virgin olive oil (1/3 cup)
- Finely chopped red onion (1/2 cup)
- Salt (1/4 tsp)
- Chopped fresh dill (1/3 cup)
- Red bell pepper, seeded and diced (1 pc, medium)
- Dijon mustard (2 tsp)
- Freshly ground pepper to taste

Instructions:

1. Whisk the mustard, pepper, lemon juice, dill, and salt in a large bowl. Whisk in the oil gradually. Add cucumber, salmon, bell pepper, onion, and lentils. Toss to coat.

2. To cook lentils, place in a saucepan and cover with water. Boil.

3. Reduce heat to a simmer and cook until it becomes just tender, or around 20 minutes for green lentils and 30mins for brown ones. Drain and rinse under cold water.

Dinner: Steamed mussels in a tomato broth

Ingredients:

- Mussels, scrubbed and debearded (3 lbs)
- Dry white wine (1 cup)
- Extra virgin olive oil (1 tsp)
- Chopped fresh parsley (2 tsp)
- Ripe plum tomatoes, cored and coarsely chopped (6 pcs)
- Garlic, finely chopped (4 cloves)

Instructions:

1. In a large pot, warm oil over low heat with a tight-fitting lid. Add garlic and cook. Stir it for around 3mins or until it becomes golden. Add the tomatoes, increase the fire to high and stir for one min more. Pour in wine and boil.

2. Add mussels, cover, steam. Give the pan a vigorous shake occasionally, until all the mussels have opened. Discard any mussels that do not open. Transfer the mussels to a serving bowl. Spoon the broth over the mussels and sprinkle with parsley.

Day 26

Breakfast: Yogurt and one pc whole wheat sliced bread

Lunch: Crunchy pear and celery salad

Ingredients:

- Raspberry, pear, cider, or other fruit vinegar
- Chopped pecans, toasted (1/2 cup)
- Butterhead or other lettuce (6 pcs, large)
- Finely diced white Cheddar cheese (1 cup)
- Honey (2 tbsp)
- Celery, trimmed and cut in half crosswise (4 stalks)
- Salt (1/4 tsp)
- Freshly ground pepper to taste
- Ripe pears, preferably Anjou or red Bartlett, diced (2 pcs)

Instructions:

1. Soak celery in a bowl of ice water for 15mins. Drain and pat dry. Cut into 1/2-in pcs.

2. Whisk the honey, sale, and vinegar in a large bowl until blended. Add pears, stir it gently to coat. Then, add cheese, celery, and pecan – stir to mix — season with pepper.

3. Divide the lettuce leaves among six plates and top with a portion of salad. Serve chilled or at room temperature.

Dinner: Vegetable Lover's chicken soup

Ingredients:

- Dry white wine (1/4 cup)
- Packed baby spinach (1 ½ cups)
- Plum tomatoes, chopped (2 pcs)
- Shallot, finely chopped (1 pc, large)
- Zucchini, finely diced (1 pc, small)
- Orzo, or other tiny pasta like farfalle (2 tbsp)
- Italian seasoning blend (1/2 tsp)
- Extra virgin olive oil (1 tbsp)
- Chicken tenders, cut into bite-size chunks (8 oz)
- Low sodium chicken broth (1 can, 14 oz)

Instructions:

1. In a large saucepan, heat oil over medium-high fire. Add chicken and cook. Stir occasionally for 3-4 mins or until it becomes brown. Transfer to a plate.

2. Add shallot, salt, Italian seasoning, and zucchini. Cook often stirring for 2-3mins or until the vegetables are slightly softened. Add broth,

tomatoes, orzo, and wine. Increase fire to high and boil while stirring occasionally.

3. Reduce heat to a simmer and cook until the pasta becomes tender or according to package directions.

4. Stir in the chicken, including the accumulated juice from it. Add spinach. Cook while stirring until the chicken is heated thoroughly.

Day 27

Breakfast: Strawberry Bruschetta

Ingredients:

- Lemon juice (2 tsp)
- Whole wheat bread (4 thick slices)
- Mascarpone (Italian cream cheese), 4 tbsp
- Grated lemon zest (1 tsp)
- Diced or sliced hulled strawberries (3 cups)
- Light brown sugar (6 tbsp)

Instructions:

1. Toast bread in a toaster.
2. Meanwhile, heat a large skillet over high heat. Add lemon zest, lemon juice, and sugar. Cook while stirring until the sugar melts and the mixture starts to bubble. Add the strawberries and stir until the juices begin to exude, and the berries are heated thoroughly.
3. Spread 1 tbsp of mascarpone on every pc or toast. Top with the warm strawberries.

Lunch: Brussels Sprouts with Lemon-Walnut Vinaigrette

Ingredients:

- Brussels sprouts, trimmed and quartered (1 lb)
- Whole grain or Dijon mustard (1 tsp)

- Minced shallot (1 tbsp)
- Lemon juice (1 tbsp)
- Freshly grated lemon zest (1/4 tsp)
- Walnut oil (2 tbsp)
- Salt (1/4 tsp)
- Freshly ground pepper to taste

Instructions:

1. Place brussels sprouts in a steamer basket and steam in a large saucepan over one inch of boiling water until it becomes tender, or around 7-8mins.

2. Meanwhile, whisk shallot, oil, mustard, lemon zest, pepper, and salt in a medium bowl. Add the sprouts to the dressing. Toss to coat.

Dinner: Mango, spinach, and avocado salad

Ingredients:

Salad

- Radicchio, torn into bite-size pcs (1 ½ cups)
- Avocado, sliced (1 pc, medium)
- Ripe mango, sliced (1 pc, small)
- Baby spinach leaves (10 cups, around 8 oz)
- Red radishes, sliced (8-12 pcs, small/1 bunch)
- Freshly ground pepper to taste

Dressing

- Dijon mustard (1 tsp)
- Red wine vinegar (1 tbsp)
- Orange juice (1/3 cup)
- Canola oil, hazelnut oil, or almond oil (2 tbsp)
- Salt (1/4 tsp)

Instructions:

1. For the dressing, whisk mustard, orange juice, oil, salt, and pepper in a bowl.

2. For the salad, just before serving, mix radishes, radicchio, spinach, and mango in a large bowl. Add the dressing and toss to coat. Garnish each serving with avocado slices.

Day 28

Breakfast: Salsa and egg toast

- Two tablespoons salsa
- One slice whole-wheat bread, toasted
- 1 large egg cooked in ¼ teaspoon olive oil or coat pan with a thin layer of cooking spray. Season with a pinch of pepper and kosher salt.

Lunch: Veggie and white bean salad

Ingredients:

- Avocado, diced (1/2 pc)
- White beans, rinsed (1/3 cup)
- Mixed greens (2 cups)
- Veggies of your choice (try tomatoes and cucumbers (3/4 cup)

Instructions:

1. Mix all ingredients and top salad with one tablespoon of red wine vinegar, freshly ground pepper, and olive oil.

Dinner: Kale with mustard and apples

Ingredients:

- Cider vinegar (2 tbsp)
- Extra virgin olive oil (1 tbsp)
- Brown sugar (2 tsp)

- Kale, ribs removed, coarsely chopped (1-1 ½ lbs)
- Whole grain mustard (4 tsp)
- Water (2/3 cup)
- Granny Smith apples, sliced (2 pcs)
- Pinch of salt

Instructions:

1. Heat oil in a Dutch oven over medium fire. Add the kale and cook. Toss with two large spoons for around 1 min or until it becomes bright green. Add water, cover, and cook. Stir it occasionally for 3mins. Stir in the apples, cover, and cook, occasionally stirring for 8-10mins or until kale becomes tender.

2. Meanwhile, whisk mustard, vinegar, salt, and brown sugar in a small bowl. Add the mixture to the kale, increasing heat to high. Boil without cover for 3-4mins or until the liquid evaporates.

Day 29

Breakfast: Tomato and egg tortilla

- Corn tortilla (1 pc)
- One large egg cooked in a ¼ teaspoon of olive oil or coat the pan with a thin layer of cooking spray. Season with a pinch of pepper.
- Five cherry tomatoes halved
- Top the tortilla with tomatoes and egg

Lunch: Scrambled eggs with smoked salmon

Ingredients:

- Heavy cream (1/2 cup)
- Sliced smoked salmon (1/4 pounds)
- Fresh chives, finely chopped (12-15 blades)
- Eggs (12 pcs)
- Freshly ground black pepper
- Salt
- Butter (2 tbsp)

Instructions:

1. Reserve 2 slices of salmon for garnish. Chop the remaining salmon into very small pcs.

2. Whisk cream and eggs together. Add ½ of chopped chives. Season eggs with pepper and salt. Preheat a large non-stick skillet over medium fire. Melt the butter in the pan and add eggs. Scramble eggs with a wooden spoon. Do not cook the eggs until dry. When eggs come together, but remain wet. Stir in the chopped salmon. Remove pan from stove and place on a trivet. Garnish the eggs with remaining chives and salmon and serve right out of the warm pan.

Dinner: Creamy Gorgonzola Polenta with Summer Squash Saute

Ingredients:

- Crumbled Gorgonzola cheese (2/3 cup)
- Vegetable broth, or low-sodium chicken broth, divided (2 cans, 14 oz)
- Zucchini halved lengthwise and sliced (2 pcs, small)
- Fresh basil, chopped (1/4 cup)
- Extra virgin olive oil (2 tbsp)
- Cornmeal (3/4 cup)
- Yellow summer squash halved lengthwise and sliced (2 pcs, small)
- Water (1 cup)
- Minced garlic (3 tbsp)

- Flour (2 tbsp)
- Freshly ground pepper (1/2 tsp)

Instructions:

4. Mix 2 and ½ broth with one cup of water in a small saucepan. Boil. Then, whisk in pepper and cornmeal slowly until smooth. Reduce fire to low, cover and cook but make sure to occasionally stir until it becomes very thick and not grainy anymore, around 10-15mins. Stir in Gorgonzola. Remove from heat.

5. Meanwhile, in a large non-stick skillet, heat oil over medium-high fire. Add garlic and cook. Stir occasionally until it starts to soften and brown in places. Sprinkle the flour over the vegetables. Stir to coat.

6. Stir in the remaining one cup broth and boil. Stir it often. Then reduce fire to medium-low and simmer. Stir occasionally until it is thickened and the vegetables become tender. Stir in the basil. Serve the saute over the polenta.

Day 30

Breakfast: Yogurt breakfast drink

Ingredients:

- Ice cubes (2 cups)
- Vanilla yogurt (2 cups)
- Peach yogurt (2 cups)
- Fat-free milk (1/2 cup)
- Thawed orange juice concentrate (1/2 cup)

Instructions:

2. In a blender, combine all ingredients except ice cubes. Cover; process until they become smooth. Add ice cubes, cover, and process again until smooth.

Lunch: Veggie-hummus sandwich

Ingredients:

- Hummus (3 tbsp)
- Cucumber slices (1/4 cup)
- Mashed avocado (1/4 cup)
- Whole wheat bread (2 slices)
- Mixed greens (1 cup)
- Red bell pepper, sliced (1/4 pcs, medium)

Instructions:

1. Spread each slice of bread with avocado and hummus. Top one slice with vegetables and press the slices together to make a sandwich.

Dinner: Corn and black bean tacos

Ingredients:

- Salsa (1/4 cup)
- Diced avocado (1/2 pc)
- Canned black beans, rinsed and mashed (1/4 cup)
- Corn (1/2 cup)
- Corn tortillas warmed (2 pcs)
- Mixed greens
- Lime juice (1 tbsp)
- Olive oil
- Pepper and kosher salt

Instructions:

1. Spread tortillas with beans. Top with salsa, corn, and avocado.

2. Top the mixed greens with olive oil, lime juice, and a pinch of pepper and kosher salt.

CHAPTER 7: STRATEGIES TO GET STARTED ON LOWER BLOOD PRESSURE MEAL DIET

While you already have a guide on the 30 superfoods to eat to lower your high blood pressure, it will be hard at first.

Lose weight

Being overweight increases the chance of developing high blood pressure. Losing weight will help not only in reducing blood pressure levels but also in preventing other diseases associated with it.

Limit alcohol intake

If you have high blood pressure and you are drinking more alcohol than the recommended intake regularly, reducing it may lower your blood pressure level up to 4 mmHg.

Do physical activities

Physical activities like aerobic activity help lower the blood pressure level because it forces the blood vessels to contract and expand. This results in keeping your blood vessels flexible.

Less salt

Cutting sodium can be hard because it is hidden in almost all foods, so it is vital to follow the meal plan strictly.

Consume more potassium

The meal plan computes the estimated amount of nutrients that you will get, and many of the meal plans daily are rich in potassium.

CHAPTER 8: OTHER LIFESTYLE CHANGES TO HELP YOU REDUCE BLOOD PRESSURE WITHOUT MEDICATION

Managing blood pressure levels is divided into 70 percent of lifestyle and 30 percent medication and prevention.

Read labels

It is hard to avoid or lower dietary sodium intake without reading the labels. While you can prepare your food using the meal plan that we shared, but it is still important to always read labels, especially when you are outside home.

Relieve stress

Stress hormones are constricting the blood vessels, and it may lead to a temporary increase in blood pressure level. It also triggers unhealthy habits like poor sleep, overeating, and more alcohol intake. Lowering stress is a priority if you want to lower blood pressure.

Exercise

It does not take much training to see the results and impact your blood pressure. You can exercise for just 30 minutes at least five days per week. These exercises may also mean doing things you love, like biking, dancing, hiking, or even daily activities like gardening.

Quit smoking

Smoking is one of the primary factors of heart disease, which is associated with high blood pressure. Since both high blood pressure and smoking increase the risk of heart complications, stopping to smoke will help reverse the risk.

Deep breathing and meditation

While meditation and deep breath fall under stress management, they deserve specific mention because they have a significant impact on lowering blood pressure. When the body is relaxed, it slows the heart rate, and thus, reduces the blood pressure level.

CONCLUSION

There are lots of people who have high blood pressure, but some of them may not even know they are included in the statistics. Eating a balanced diet and leading a healthy lifestyle results in keeping your blood pressure levels in check. The snacks and meals in this book follow a high-blood pressure solution and prevention eating pattern.

The meal plan provides the nutrients the body needs to function correctly with a specific amount to not only manage blood pressure but also prevent other associated diseases from developing and help you lose weight, too.

It only proves that making changes to diet and lifestyle is the best way to control high blood pressure without taking any medications. Medications that reduce blood pressure tend to work well, but they are not necessarily attacking the cause of the problem. Thus, a high blood pressure solution diet plan is an effective first-line defense for prevention and management.

FINAL WORDS

Thank you again for purchasing this book!

We hope this book can help you.

The next step is for you to **join our email newsletter** to receive updates on any upcoming new book releases or promotions. You can sign-up for free, and as a bonus, you will also receive our "*7 Fitness Mistakes You Don't Know You're Making*" book! This bonus book breaks down many of the most common fitness mistakes and will demystify many of the complexities and science of getting into shape. Having all this fitness knowledge and science organized into an actionable step-by-step book will help you get started in the right direction in your fitness journey! To join our free email newsletter and grab your free book, please visit the link and signup: **www.effingopublishing.com/gift**

Finally, if you enjoyed this book, then we would like to ask you for a favor, would you be kind enough to leave a review for this book? It would be much appreciated! **Thank you, and good luck on your journey!**

ABOUT THE CO-AUTHOR

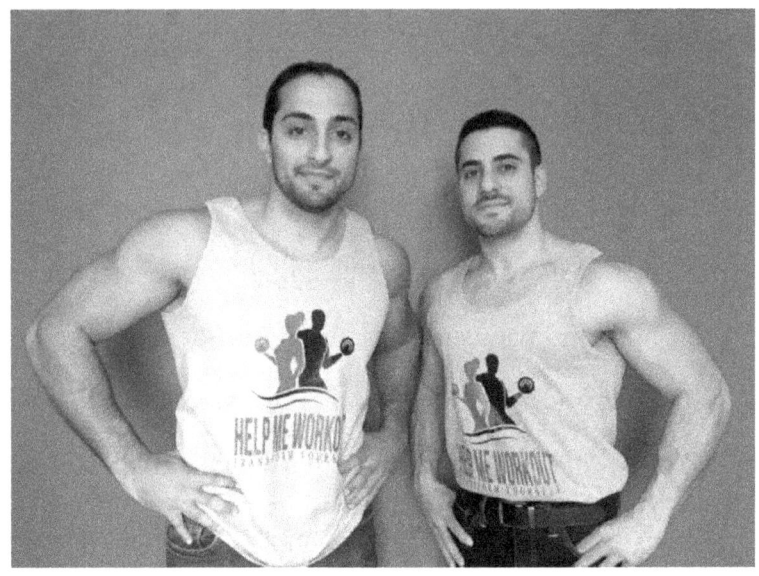

Our name is Alex & George Kaplo; we're both certified personal trainers from Montreal, Canada. We will start by saying we are not the biggest guys you will ever meet, and this has never really been our goal. We started working out to overcome our biggest insecurity when we were younger, which was our self-confidence. You may be going through some challenges right now, or you may simply want to get fit, and we can certainly relate.

We always kind were interested in the health & fitness world and wanted to gain some muscle due to the numerous bullying in our teenage years. We figured we could do something about how our body looks like. This was the beginning of our transformation journey. We had no idea where to start, but we both just got started. We felt worried and afraid at times that other people would make fun of us for doing the exercises the wrong way. We always wished we had a friend to guide us and who could just show us the ropes.

After a lot of work, studying, and countless trials and errors. Some people began to notice how we were both getting more fit and how we were starting to form a keen interest in the topic. This led many friends and new faces to come to us and ask us for fitness advice. At first, it seemed odd when people asked us to help them get in shape. But what kept us going is when they started to see changes in their own body and told us it's the first time that they saw real results! From there, more people kept coming to us, and it made both of us realize after so much reading and studying in this field that it did help us, but it also allowed us to help others. To date, we have coached and trained numerous clients who have achieved some pretty amazing results.

Today, both of us own & operate this publishing business, where we bring passionate and expert authors to write about health and fitness topics. We also run an online fitness business, and we would love to connect with you by inviting you to visit the website on the following page and signing up for our e-mail newsletter (you will even get a free book).

Last but not least, if you are in the position we were once in and you want some guidance, don't hesitate and ask... I will be there to help you out!

Your coaches,

Alex & George Kaplo

Download another book for Free

We want to thank you for purchasing this book and offer you another book (just as long and valuable as this book), "Health & Fitness Mistakes You Don't Know You're Making," completely free.

Visit the link below to signup and receive it:

www.effingopublishing.com/gift

In this book, we will break down the most common health & fitness mistakes, you are probably committing right now, and will reveal how you can quickly get in the best shape of your life!

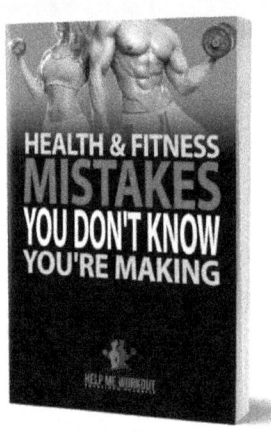

In addition to this valuable gift, you will also have an opportunity to get our new books for free, enter giveaways, and receive other useful emails from us. Again, visit the link to sign up:

www.effingopublishing.com/gift

Copyright 2019 by Effingo Publishing - All Rights Reserved.

This document by Effingo Publishing, owned by the A&G Direct Inc company, is geared towards providing exact and reliable information in regards to the topic and issue covered. The publication is sold with the idea that the publisher is not required to render accounting, officially permitted or otherwise qualified services. If advice is necessary, legal or professional, a practiced individual in the profession should be ordered.

From a Declaration of Principles which was accepted and approved equally by a Committee of the American Bar Association and a Committee of Publishers and Associations.

In no way is it legal to reproduce, duplicate, or transmit any part of this document in either electronic means or printed format. Recording of this publication is strictly prohibited, and any storage of this document is not allowed unless with written permission from the publisher. All rights reserved.

The information provided herein is stated to be truthful and consistent, in that any liability, in terms of inattention or otherwise, by any usage or abuse of any policies, processes, or directions contained within is the solitary and utter responsibility of the recipient reader. Under no circumstances will any legal responsibility or blame be held against the publisher for any reparation, damages, or monetary loss due to the information herein, either directly or indirectly.

The information herein is offered for informational purposes solely and is universal as so. The presentation of the data is without a contract or any type of guarantee assurance.

The trademarks that are used are without any consent, and the publication of the trademark is without permission or backing by the trademark owner. All trademarks and brands within this book are for clarifying purposes only and are owned by the owners themselves, not affiliated with this document.

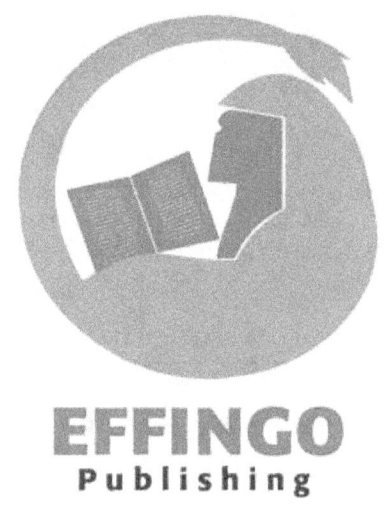

For more great books, visit:

EffingoPublishing.com

www.ingramcontent.com/pod-product-compliance
Lightning Source LLC
LaVergne TN
LVHW011710060526
838200LV00051B/2850